# Conversations in the Disciplines:
## Sustaining Rural Populations

edited by

*Lindsay Lake Morgan*

and

*Pamela Stewart Fahs*

Global Academic Publishing
Binghamton University
2007

Copyright © 2007

All rights reserved. No portion of this publication may be duplicated in any way without the express written consent of the publisher, except in the form of brief excerpts of quotations for the purposes of review.

Library of Congress Cataloging-in-Publication Data

Conversations in the disciplines : sustaining rural populations / edited by Lindsay Lake Morgan and Pamela Stewart Fahs.
   p. ; cm.
  Papers from a conference held April 2004 at Binghamton University.
  Includes bibliographical references.
  ISBN-13: 978-1-58684-269-7 (pbk. : alk. paper)
  ISBN-10: 1-58684-269-2 (pbk. : alk. paper)
  1. Rural health services--Congresses. I. Morgan, Lindsay Lake. II. Fahs, Pamela Stewart. III. State University of New York at Binghamton.
  [DNLM: 1. Rural Health Services--Congresses. 2. Community Health Nursing--Congresses. 3. Rural Health--Congresses. 4. Rural Population--Congresses. WA 390 C766 2007]
   RA771.A2C66 2007
   362.1'04257--dc22
                                       2007017296

Decker School of Nursing
Binghamton University
PO Box 6000
Binghamton, NY 13902
607-777-2311

This monograph was published with support from
the *Decker School of Nursing* by

Global Academic Publishing
Harpur College Dean's Office
Binghamton University, LNG99
Binghamton, New York 13902-6000
Phone: (607) 777-4495; Fax: (607) 777-6132
Email: gap@binghamton.edu
Website: http://academicpublishing.binghamton.edu

# Contents

| | |
|---|---|
| Acknowledgements | *v* |
| Contributing Authors | *vii* |
| Foreword | *xi* |

CHAPTER 1
    Keynote Address: Rural Healthy People 2010 and     *1*
    Sustaining Rural Populations
        *Larry Gamm*

CHAPTER 2
    Collaboration in Rural School Health     *13*
        *Laura R. Bronstein and Susan Terwilliger*

CHAPTER 3
    A Community Action Mandate for Oral Health in     *31*
    Rural Populations
        *Sarah Hall Gueldner, Carolyn Pierce, Peter Beatty,*
        *Frederick J. Lacey, Lynne B. Lacey, Leann Lesperance,*
        *Joyce Hyatt, Fran Srnka-Debnar, Susan Terwilliger,*
        *and Lucy Bianco*

CHAPTER 4
    Health Maintenance Flow Sheet for Agricultural Workers     *53*
        *Lindsay Lake Morgan*

CHAPTER 5
    Sustaining Geriatric Rural Populations     *63*
        *John A. Krout and Marilyn Kinner*

CHAPTER 6
    Meeting the Rural Nursing Shortage Needs:     *75*
    An Evening/Weekend Nursing Program
        *Claire Ligeikis-Clayton*

CHAPTER 7
    Using the Concepts of the Nursing Paradigm to     *85*
    Sustain Rural Populations
        *Carolyn Pierce*

CHAPTER 8
    Quality of Life in Rural Women with Heart Failure:     *97*
    The State of the Science
        *Carolyn Pierce*

CHAPTER 9
    Notification of Eligibility for Hospice Services for    111
    Terminally Ill Pulmonary Disease, End-Stage
    Renal Disease, and Amyotrophic Lateral
    Sclerosis Inpatients at a University Hospital
            *Melanie Kalman and Roberta Rolland*
CHAPTER 10
    Sexual Behavior Patterns of Rural Men who    123
    Have Sex with Men: Description and
    Implications for Intervention
            *Anthony R. D'Augelli, Deborah Bray Preston,*
            *Richard E. Cain, and Frederick W. Schulze*
CHAPTER 11
    Measurement in Rural Research:    149
    Matching the Instrument to the Population
            *Janet Ambrogne Sobczak*
CHAPTER 12
    Barriers to Research Participation Identified by    161
    Rural People
            *Lindsay Lake Morgan, Pamela Stewart Fahs,*
            *and Jamie Klesh*

# Acknowledgements

In April 2004 a conference entitled Conversations in the Disciplines: Sustaining Rural Populations was held at Binghamton University. This monograph is one outcome of that conference.

Our thanks go to the Office of the Provost of the State University of New York in Albany who supported the initial grant for the Conversations in the Disciplines conference. The four collaborating partners for the conference included: Pamela Stewart Fahs as Director of the O'Connor Office of Rural Health Studies, Decker School of Nursing and Robin Russel, Director of the Division of Social Work, in the School of Education & Human Development of Binghamton University; Claire Ligeikis Clayton, Chair of the Department of Nursing of Broome Community College; and David Brown, Director of the Polson Institute for Global Development, College of Agriculture & Life Science of Cornell University. The conference was also fiscally supported by the Decker School of Nursing, Binghamton University; the Polson Institute for Global Development at Cornell University, and Zeta Iota Chapter of Sigma Theta Tau, the International Nursing Honor Society. In addition, Dr. Gale Spencer provided 20 scholarships to the conference for community health nursing students and their clinical preceptors, through the Community Health Nursing Masters Program Expansion Grant. Dr. Gary James of the Institute of Primary and Preventive Health Care (IPPH) was supportive by providing personnel to assist in the production of the conference. A special thank you goes to Ann Casella who was instrumental in making the conference a successful one with her dedication and work.

There were many, many individuals, students, staff, faculty and administrators of the Decker School of Nursing who were instrumental in making Conversations in the Disciplines: Sustaining Rural Populations a successful conference, to each of you "Thank You." This assistance has continued as we have undertaken the task of editing this monograph. During this time, Dean Joyce Ferrario has provided encouragement and support.

To all who have contributed chapters to this monograph, our heartfelt thanks. Your work and words will add to the science of rural health. It is our hope that this is just the beginning, not the end of the conversation on sustaining rural populations.

# Contributing Authors

**Peter Beatty, PhD**
New York State AHEC System
SUNY Upstate Medical University, Syracuse, NY

**Lucy Bianco, RDH**
Lourdes Center for Oral Health
Binghamton, NY

**Laura Bronstein, LCSW-R, ACSW, PhD**
Department of Social Work, College of Community and Public Affairs
Binghamton University, State University of New York

**Richard E. Cain, PhD**
Department of Health Education
Rhode Island College
Providence, RI

**Anthony R. D'Augelli, PhD**
Department of Human Development and Family Studies
The Pennsylvania State University
University Park, PA

**Pamela Stewart Fahs, RN, DSN**
Decker School of Nursing
Binghamton University, State University of New York

**Larry Gamm, PhD**
Southwest Rural Health Research Center, School of Rural Public Health
Texas A&M University System Health Science Center
Bryan, TX

**Sarah Hall Gueldner, DSN, RN, FAAN, FGSA**
Frances Payne Bolton School of Nursing
Case Western Reserve University and
Decker School of Nursing
Binghamton University, State University of New York

**Joyce Hyatt, PhD, PCNP**
Health Ministry of the Southern Tier
Corning, NY

**Melanie Kalman, PhD, CNS**
College of Nursing
SUNY Upstate Medical University, Syracuse, NY

**Marilyn Kinner**
Ithaca College Gerontology Institute
Ithaca, NY

**Jamie Klesh, MS, APRN, PhD Student**
Decker School of Nursing
Binghamton University, State University of New York

**John A. Krout, PhD**
Ithaca College Gerontology Institute
Ithaca, NY

**Frederick J. Lacey, DMD, PLLC**
Private Practice, Binghamton, NY

**Lynne B. Lacey, RDH, MS**
Dental Hygienist, Binghamton, NY

**Leann Lesperance, MD, PhD, FAAP**
Watson School of Engineering & Applied Science
Binghamton University, State University of New York and
Department of Pediatrics, SUNY Upstate Medical University

**Claire Ligeikis-Clayton, RN, EdD**
Department of Nursing
Broome Community College
Binghamton, NY

**Lindsay Lake Morgan, PhD, RN, GNP**
Decker School of Nursing
Binghamton University, State University of New York

**Carolyn Pierce, DSN, RN**
Decker School of Nursing and
Watson School of Engineering and Applied Science
Binghamton University, State University of New York

**Deborah Bray Preston, PhD, RN**
School of Nursing
The Pennsylvania State University
University Park, PA

**Roberta Rolland, MS, RN**
Upstate Medical University Hospital, Syracuse, NY

**Frederick W. Schulze, D Ed**
Department of Health Science
Lock Haven University of Pennsylvania
Lock Haven, PA

**Janet Ambrogne Sobczak, RN, PhD**
Decker School of Nursing
Binghamton University, State University of New York

**Fran Srnka-Debnar, MS, RN**
Decker School of Nursing
Binghamton University, State University of New York

**Susan Terwilliger, MS, RNCS, PNP**
Decker School of Nursing
Binghamton University, State University of New York

# Foreword

**PAMELA STEWART FAHS**
*Decker Chair in Rural Nursing*

As clinicians, researchers, and educators who work with people in rural areas, we know well the problems confronting rural populations. Perhaps we even know the problems too well. Our work in the past has often focused on the identification and description of the issues and barriers to health faced by rural dwellers. The Conversations program of the State University of New York is designed to bring together members of the State University of New York faculty and visiting scholars for conferences that cross campus borders. The purposes of this conference series included a means to facilitate the examination of trends and research in a topical area; and to spur professional development both across and within disciplines. The disciplines of Nursing, Anthropology, Social Science, and Social Work came together at this Conversations in the Disciplines conference in April 2004 to examine research and programs targeting rural populations. We learned from our colleagues within and across disciplines. Conversations in the Disciplines: Sustaining Rural Populations met the objectives of the Conversations program with a well planned and executed meeting. Four disciplines from three different campuses came together for the planning and grant application to support this conference. Conference participants represented academia, health care providers and professionals in the health and human services arena. Dr. Lindsay Morgan, co-editor, and myself are pleased to bring you this monograph that presents several of the presented papers for those people who did not have an opportunity to attend. This monograph builds upon that initial work with papers that go beyond those presented at the conference, some of these papers had their initial work begun because of papers presented at the conference, others were reviewed and added as people heard about the conference and wanted to contribute to the work in progress.

The conference Keynote Speaker, Larry Gamm, PhD of the Southwest Rural Health Research Center, School of Rural Public Health at Texas A&M, focused the conference with examples of programs that have been most successful in sustaining rural populations. These programs often pull from ideas of disease prevention, health promotion, or chronic disease management. Although they recognize limited resources, synergy is gained by building upon community partnerships to produce programs that go beyond describing problems and issues of rural living to those that strive to sustain rural populations. Day one of the conference began with symposia which varied from information and educational technologies, to social and economic change in rural America, and into diagnosing and managing Alzheimer's Disease in rural populations. Joyce Ferrario, PhD reviewed the state of the science of rural nursing by discussing the very stimulating topics emerging from dissertations from the first PhD program in Rural Nursing in the country, offered here at Binghamton University. In this monograph you will be able to read the work of those conducting research and addressing health issues in rural populations. Conference topics ranged from subject recruitment to instrument development and data analysis using statistical modeling. The topic of collaboration in rural settings allowed attendees to explore the areas of multidisciplinary collaborations, the use of telemedicine in rural outreach programs, and collaboration in rural school health. Health and safety topics included the discussion of food systems, use of a screening tool among agricultural workers, and respiratory conditions among farmers. Day one ended with an enticing poster session where work in progress and a variety of rural research and community projects could be viewed.

Day two began with round table discussions. This breakfast event allowed individuals from different disciplines working on similar issues to come together and explore common ground, learn from the leaders in the field, and build networks and relationships between and among those whose work focuses on sustaining rural populations. Day two sessions covered a wide range of topics including cardiovascular health in rural populations, sustaining rural emergency medical services, preparing professionals and paraprofessionals to meet the needs of rural health care systems. Rural populations by age were explored in sessions that focused on school aged, adolescents, adults, and geriatric populations. Conversations

*Foreword*

in the Disciplines: Sustaining Rural Populations will be remembered as a forum that moved us forward in our work with rural populations.

This monograph explores issues of theory, research, and practice. These readings reflect the state of the science of rural health care as well as puts forth calls to action for sustaining and enhancing health for rural populations. I believe the monograph, *Conversations in the Disciplines: Sustaining Rural Populations,* will be helpful to you the reader as you work to promote health among rural dwellers in the effort to sustain rural populations.

*Chapter 1*

# Keynote Address:
## *Rural Healthy People 2010 and Sustaining Rural Populations*

### LARRY GAMM

**Abstract:** This paper summarizes my keynote presentation to the Conversations in the Disciplines: Sustaining Rural Populations symposium in April 2004 at Binghamton University. The presentation was designed to reflect the contribution of our Southwest Rural Health Research Center work titled "Rural Healthy People 2010 — A Companion Document to Healthy People 2010" and our related work on disease management to the theme of the conference on sustaining rural populations. Accepting that challenge, the presentation is outlined as follows. First, a number of rural health disparities are identified in Rural Health People 2010. Second, an underlying condition of rural disadvantage with respect to many health conditions is limited access to care. Third, given limited access to care, it is all the more important that there be a "meeting in the middle" of community health, in the form of disease prevention and health promotion, and chronic disease management. Finally, given limited infrastructure and other resources in many rural areas, care coordination efforts supported by community health partnerships are important for sustaining rural populations.

## Introduction

The purpose of Rural Healthy People 2010 is to identify rural health priorities among Healthy People 2010's 28 focus areas and summarize rural health research and models of rural practice for addressing rural health priorities. A closely related purpose is to attract more rural people to the impressive resources offered by Rural Healthy People 2010. I should point out that just a glimpse of total Rural

Healthy People 2010 efforts and products are presented here without footnotes. The bibliography at the end include articles describing the process and the easy access to three volumes that present both summaries of rural health research literature and models for practice associated with over one-dozen rural health priorities.

The first steps in Rural Healthy People 2010 was to conduct a survey of rural health leaders to establish rural health priorities and to begin the process of nominating models for practice, i.e., successful efforts pursued by rural communities to address these priorities. Over 500 state and local rural health leaders responded to the nationwide survey including: (a) state leaders from state offices of rural health, state primary care offices and associations, and state rural health associations; (b) local rural public health agencies; (c) rural health clinics and community health centers; and (d) rural hospitals. Each of the groups were asked to check five of the 28 Healthy People 2010 goals that they considered the highest priority in rural health. Based on the average of the responses for each group, the four groups of leaders produced the following ranking of the top sixteen rural health priorities (see Table 1).

**Table 1**
*A Ranking of the Rural Health Priorities*

| Rank | Healthy People 2010 Goals |
|---|---|
| 1 | Access to Quality Health Care |
| 2 | Heart Disease and Stroke |
| 2 | Diabetes |
| 4 | Mental Health and Mental Disorders |
| 5 | Oral Health |
| 6 | Tobacco Use |
| 6 | Substance Abuse |
| 6 | Education and Community-Based Programs |
| 6 | Maternal, Infant, and Child Health |
| 10 | Nutrition and Overweight |
| 10 | Cancer |
| 10 | Public Health Infrastructure |
| 13 | Immunization and Infectious Disease |
| 13 | Injury and Violence Prevention |

The survey also produced over 300 nominations for Models for Practice (MFP) corresponding to the priorities. Rural Healthy People 2010 investigated these and other nominations to produce over 80 MFP, demonstrating successful community level action to address these priorities. The MFPs appear on the Southwest Rural Health Research Center's website and correspond to all of the priorities reviewed there. The bank of MFPs is searchable by topic area and by state location of the MFP. For each, a general blue print is presented first, outlining what the MFP does and how to address the target rural health need. Then, evidence is provided to reflect outcomes and impacts associated with efforts. This is followed by a review of the origins of the MFP, followed by a review of the challenges and barriers faced by the MFP stakeholders and the strategies and action they employed to overcome them. Each MFP concludes with the MFP's contact person's identification and contact information.

Several summary observations flowed out of reviewing the research literature and MFPs for many of these rural health priorities. First, one cannot generalize to all rural areas. For example, rural areas differ widely in the degree to which they reflect health disparities in relation to urban areas or the larger nation. There is, nonetheless, substantial evidence that health conditions and access to providers and insurance are poorer among many rural areas. At the same time, MFPs offer evidence from many disadvantaged rural areas of the pursuit of local solutions and advocacy for policy change. Viewed more broadly, Rural Healthy People 2010 suggests that the state of rural health finds "the glass is both half full and half empty." This is reflected in a brief examination of findings associated with two health conditions and selected MFPs.

## Diabetes

Diabetes has been termed a national epidemic. It is the sixth leading cause of death and the sixth or seventh cause of hospitalization among men and women, 45 and older. There are higher diabetes rates among Hispanics and African Americans than Caucasians. Despite the tradition of referring to Type 2 diabetes as adult-onset diabetes, it is being diagnosed increasingly among teenagers and even younger children. Somewhat prevalent among populations in the Southwest and Southeast, diabetes is also associated with obesity and relatively more sedentary lifestyles, two other conditions addressed within Rural Healthy People 2010.

Among several MFPs addressing diabetes is that of Pennsylvania's Laurel Health System and the associated Tioga County Partnership for Community Health. Identifying diabetes as a local health priority through a community survey in 1992, the Partnership undertook community-wide diabetes patient education. A few year's later the Laurel Health Systems' Federally Qualified Health Centers (FQHCs) began participation in the National Diabetes Collaborative sponsored by the U.S. Bureau of Primary Health Care and demonstrated a profound impact on successful management of diabetes. The partnership, working under a state grant, facilitated collaboration of FQHCs with other primary care physician practices in this rural county to ensure the widespread inclusion of diabetics in a local registry and adoption of appropriate diabetes management practices.

Two other MFPs reflected a broader strategy that embraced diabetes detection and management among other targets. An 11-county Mississippi Delta Partnership of many state and local partner organizations demonstrated success in addressing hypertension and diabetes among African Americans, age 55 and younger. Another MFP was undertaken by the South Carolina Geriatric Partnership which worked through FQHCs. This group undertook screening, including diabetes, and primary care and offered transportation, case management, and services eligibility screening for elderly African American poor.

## Mental Health and Substance Abuse

Mental health and substance abuse, like oral health and diabetes, are receiving increasing attention as rural health priorities. The research literature suggests that rural people are less likely to pursue mental health services and have higher suicide rates. Rural youth reflect higher rates of use of alcohol, methamphetamines, and inhalants. In addition to the high toll such maladies manifest by themselves, the dual diagnosis of depression or other mental illness and substance abuse is often highly resistant to intervention. Depression, for example, is often identified as a significant "co-morbidity" among those suffering from congestive heart failure (CHF), diabetes, or obesity.

Among a number of mental health and/or substance abuse MFPs is a recently developed behavioral health department program in a Sumpter County, Florida FQHC that participates in a U.S. Bureau of Primary Health Care sponsored depression collaborative. Another MFP is located in Sitka, Alaska where Community Family Services supports village providers, paraprofessionals, who are cross trained in mental and substance abuse and are backed up by clinicians. Still a third is based in Marshfield, Wisconsin and serves both Caucasian and several minority groups, e.g., American Indians and Hmong, in rural counties through a youth development and substance abuse prevention effort.

## Community Health Intervention and Medical Care

Both diabetes and behavioral health are addressed by MFPs that often address a combination of effective community health intervention and medical care. More generally, it appears that a number of rural health providers and rural community partnerships recognize the need to address both community health and medical care to effectively address the heath needs of patients and advance the health status of the larger population. More generally, they reflect a convergence between public health and medical care. See Figure 1.

**Figure 1**
*Public Health and Medical Care*

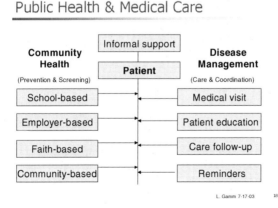

In Figure 1, the community health side concentrates on reducing the number of patients by effective prevention efforts, on early identification of health problems to increase patient access to necessary care, and reinforcing positive health activities among patients who have undergone treatment. On the right hand side, disease management promotes a coordinated set of steps that engage the patient's participation in all stages of care, recovery, and health maintenance. Effective interventions on both the community health side and disease management side recognize the need to "meet in middle" to support the health education effort by engaging the informal support systems for individuals participating in prevention programs or the disease management effort for patients whose treatment and health is to be optimized.

On the community health side, sustaining rural populations will require increased reliance of evidence-based prevention programs with students, employees, community organization participants, and the public. Ideally, there will be evidence of a community partnership on agreed upon chronic disease prevention goals. On the medical care side, sustaining rural populations will require health care plans and providers, public and private, to emphasize effective management of chronic illness in leadership, benefits packages, and provider incentives.

Activities from both sides must attend to the central role of individual and social support of students, workers, and patients who are to benefit from community health or medical care interventions. On the medical care side, the centrality of the patient role in care relationships must be recognized as must be the role of informal caregivers and families. On the community side and medical care side, attention must be given to building and maintaining a cultural "connection" in prevention and in patient care. Such connections are especially important in building knowledge for informed decisions and trust and overcoming doubts, fears, or stigma that patients, families, or community groups might associate with various illnesses.

## *Disease Management in Rural Communities*

Many of the issues raised in the preceding discussion address the need for effective disease management (DM), including reaching out to patients who may need support from their families, employers, and others. Another study within the Southwest Rural Health Research Center has addressed the activities of health providers and/or health plans associated with six rural health systems across the country.

Based on survey results from 71 DM participants, DM leaders (15%), DM nurses (45%), and DM physicians (40%), a number of advantages and disadvantages for support of DM activities were identified within rural areas. A number of relative advantages are presented in Figure 2. Several advantages may suggest that in rural settings with relatively greater travel distances to medical facilities, rural patients and their families place greater value on the convenience and assurance associated with DM.

**Figure 2**
*Rural Advantages in Disease Management*

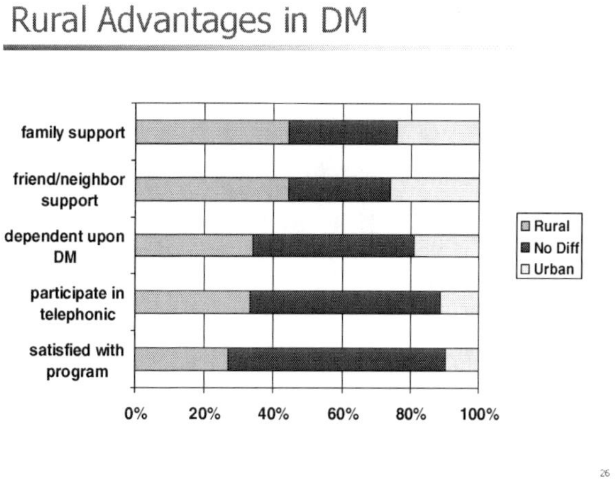

### Rural Advantages in DM

[Bar chart showing Rural, No Diff, and Urban responses across categories: family support, friend/neighbor support, dependent upon DM, participate in telephonic, satisfied with program; x-axis 0% to 100%]

DM participants also point to a number of relative disadvantages that may confront rural participants in DM, see Figure 3. The disadvantages generally revolve around less access to services, e.g., lab, pharmacy, or social services that may be deemed necessary to supporting effective DM.

More generally, professionals participating in DM in the six rural systems suggest that DM is not for everyone. Only an estimated 55% to 64% of patients in the DM programs comply with DM program instructions. The combination of advantages and disadvantages in reaching rural DM patients suggest that additional needs for tactics for encouraging patient participation in DM are needed; counseling, social support, or incentives to overcome non-responsive attitudes and behaviors by patients; access to supportive providers and ancillary medical and social services; and assistance that can address financial impediments, such as drug costs; and distance and weather factors.

**Figure 3**
*Rural Disadvantages in Disease Management*

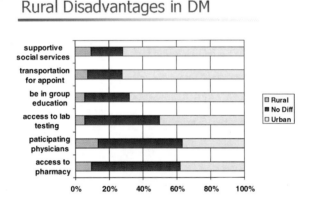

## Policy Implications for Sustaining Rural Populations

Sustaining rural people calls for moving beyond traditional disease management to care coordination and case management and to community health serving multiple rural populations. At a minimum, it is critical to move beyond disease specific coordination — among health plans and providers to better coordinate and extend care to patients with multiple co-morbidities. Although DM has been successful in some settings in penetrating and coordinating what are sometime separate health provider silos, DM is often less successful in coordinating care across several illness categories (see Figure 4).

Among the existing approaches that offer additional support for coordinating care across diagnoses and organizations are community health nursing and community-oriented primary care (COPC) supported by population-health models, community needs assessments, and community health partnerships. Although the models serve to bridge illnesses and medical and community health approaches, they are seldom fully supported.

**Figure 4**
*Silos and Tunnels in Disease Management*

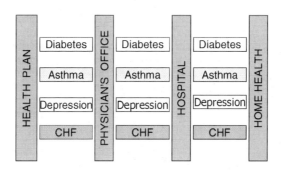

DM must be more than "savings" or "profits." DM strategies should serve the health of patients by enabling patients and providers. That is, patients must be more fully engaged in partnering in their own treatment and providers must be enabled to call upon the support of informal caregivers and other organizations in the community. DM strategies, emphasizing information technologies and social technologies, must increasingly reach across all rural populations.

Health policy at all levels, should consider health plan, provider, and community options for DM sponsorship and delivery. Medicaid experiments in several states support private DM company approaches. Also, other arrangements similar to regional and community DM efforts in a few Medicaid programs might be expanded.

Consideration should be given to regional and community-based DM providers for "selected populations" and paid by public and private insurers, providers, and state and local agencies.

As attention is focused on improved linkages between community health and disease management, simultaneous engagement of health providers and other community level organizations is called for. Figure 5 suggests the kind of resource bridging that may be necessary across a number of community institutions to build and sustain a nexus between community health and disease management.

**Figure 5**
*Resources Bridging*

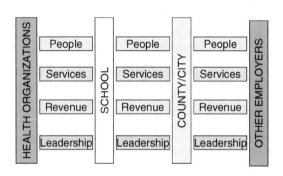

Rural Healthy People 2010 reflects impressive creativity on the part of rural communities and their organizations. Rural agencies, providers and community partnerships often offer "Make Do" strategies even as they advocate for more systematic support from state and federal agencies and private health insurers and providers. Many of these strategies include as essential components, health promotion, prevention, and care management strategies that sustain rural populations. Policy-makers must look at such models and consider how policies and programs can support evaluation, sustainability, and replication of effective options in rural areas. Many of these models for practice face the common challenges of funding and stretching local resources. At the same time, many of them are rich in professional and community stewardship and policy advocacy.

## BIBLIOGRAPHY

Bolin, J., & Gamm, L. (2003). Chronic disease management in rural areas. *Southwest Rural Health Research Center Newsletter*, 1(3), 1–2.

Gamm, L. & Hutchison, L. (2003). Rural health priorities in America: Where you stand depends on where you sit. *Journal of Rural Health*, 19(3), 209–213.

Gamm, L. & Hutchison, L. (2004). Rural healthy people 2010: Evolving interactive practice. *American Journal of Public Health*, 94(10), 1711–1712.

Gamm, L. & Hutchison, L. (Eds.) (2004, 2005) *Rural healthy people 2010: A companion document to healthy people 2010*. Vol 3. College Station, Texas: School of Rural Public Health, Texas A&M University System Health Science Center. www.srph.tamhsc.edu/centers/rhp2010

Gamm, L., Hutchison, L., Dabney, B. & Dorsey, A. (Eds). (2003). *Rural healthy people 2010: A companion document to healthy people 2010*. Vols. 1 & 2. College Station, Texas: School of Rural Public Health, Texas A&M University System Health Science Center. www.srph.tamhsc.edu/centers/rhp2010

*Chapter 2*

# Collaboration in Rural School Health

### LAURA R. BRONSTEIN AND SUSAN TERWILLIGER

## Rural School Health

There are various definitions of rural school communities. Some use population size of less than 2,500 persons (Ricketts, 1999), some use population density of less than ten persons per square mile (Winstead-Fry, 1992), and some consider proximity to metropolitan areas (Rural Assistance Center, 2004). The National Middle School Association combines the definitions of rural and small schools to mean schools in a rural or small town setting with a population of less than 25,000 persons (Rural Assistance Center, 2004). Using this definition, the Mid-continent Research for Education and Learning (McREL) Initiative identifies that 24.6 percent of America's school age children are educated in rural schools. Using stricter criteria, over seven million children, or one in six, attend a school in a rural community of less than 2,500 persons (Arnold, 2004).

### *Rural Communities*

Rural communities have different health care strengths and challenges (Long & Weinert, 1992). Compared to metropolitan communities, rural areas often have a larger elderly population, lower household income, higher poverty rates, higher unemployment rates, and more persons with less education. Transportation and community services are often scarce. In addition, there are higher rates of chronic illness, infant mortality, and injuries (Ricketts, 1999). Rural populations are more likely to describe their health as fair or poor and their health care services as limited and less accessible. Other factors include: (a) present time orientation where health beliefs are tied to ability to work; (b) isolation due to distance, independency and pride as well as self reliance; (c) more discrimination in developing and maintaining social affiliations; (d) hesitancy to accept outsider help; and (e) concerns about less anonymity (Green-Hernandez, 1992). Top rural health concerns are: (a) access to services; (b) diseases of cancer, diabetes, heart disease, and stroke; (c) maternal, infant and child well-being; (d) mental health and mental disorders; (e) lifestyle behaviors of nutrition, weight, physical activity, and substance and tobacco use; and (f) oral health care (Gamm, Hutchison, Dabney, & Dorsey, 2003a, 2003b). Health care services in rural areas have unique challenges.

## School Health

Schools are important institutions. They are second only to homes as places that children spend their time. Schools often play a prominent role in communities in terms of activities and services. The Centers for Disease Control and Prevention (CDC) describes the coordinated school health model as an ideal (CDC & Coordinating Center for Health Promotion, 2007). This model includes eight components and requires significant collaborations. The components include: (a) health education; (b) physical education; (c) health services; (d) nutrition services; (e) health promotion for staff; (f) counseling, psychological, and social services; (g) a healthy environment; and (h) family and community involvement. Important partners include: (a) students, (b) families, (c) administrators, (d) teachers, (e) nurses, (f) home-school coordinators, (g) psychologists, (h) social workers, (i) environmental health and safety workers, (j) community agencies and businesses, and (k) local and state legislators.

Schools are also important players in meeting the Healthy People 2010 goals for children and youth. The critical objectives related to this population focus around the areas of chronic illness, mental health, preventable injuries, responsible sexual behavior, substance abuse including tobacco use, and violence (Krause, O'Sullivan, Terwilliger, & Nierstedt, 2004). The CDC illuminates the critical need and promising practices for effective school health programs to achieve the objectives of Healthy People 2010 (CDC & Health Resources and Services Administration [HRSA], 2004). Promising practices for school health programs include coordinating multiple components and multiple strategies, coordinating the activities of agencies and organizations whose goal is to improve children and youth health status, implementing the CDC school health guidelines, and using a program planning process. The eight priority actions center around monitoring critical health-related behaviors; establishing partnerships, policies and dedicated support for school health at the state level; developing plans to provide professional development opportunities while increasing awareness of the health and academic needs of this population; and evaluating and improving programs on a regular basis.

CDC and HRSA have identified three target outcomes specific to the elementary, middle, and high school settings: (a) increase high school completion from 85% to 90%; (b) increase the proportion of middle, junior high, and senior high schools that provide school health education to prevent health problems from 28% to 70%; and (c) increase the proportion of schools that have a school nurse-to-student ratio of 1:750 from 28% to 50% (CDC & HRSA, 2004). Dropping out is associated with multiple social and health problems with some symptoms evident in early grades: (a) low academic achievement, (b) more than a year behind in grade level, and (c) chronic truancy. Health education needs to focus on critical areas for the school age population such as unhealthy dietary patterns, inadequate physical education and high rates of unintentional injuries.

Nurses have been in schools for over 100 years (Ihlenfeld, 2004). Initially, school nurses focused on communicable disease and absenteeism. Today, school nurses provide and coordinate physical health, mental health, and social services for all children. In addition, more children with special needs are included in the classrooms requiring the school nurse to supervise daily medications, high technology procedures and special diets.

At the national level the National Coordinating Committee on School Health (NCCSH) was established in 1994 by the Secretaries of the Departments of Education, Health and Human Services, and Agriculture. There are now 75 members on the committee. In addition, CDC's Division of Adolescent and School Health (DASH) provides fiscal and technical support to national, state, and local organizations. Since schools receive much of their funding from the state, CDC DASH also encourages state partnerships for coordinated school health programs and professional development consortiums. Finally, CDC DASH has developed numerous tools and resources to improve school health programs that can be utilized at the local level. (Fisher et al., 2003).

## *School-Based Health Centers*

A promising model for collaboration in school health, in addition to traditional school nursing and counseling services, is the School-Based Health Center (SBHC). Developed in the last 30 years, SBHCs provide mental health, counseling and substance abuse treatment; health supervision, screenings, physical examinations and immunizations; and urgent care services (Pastore & Techow, 2004). As of 1998, 1157 SBHCs existed in America's 110,000 schools with 26% in rural schools (Center for Health and Health Care in Schools, 2004). Nurses, health educators, primary care providers including nurse practitioners, physicians and physician assistants, and mental health providers such as clinical social workers, psychologists, and psychiatrists staff SBHCs. Thirty-eight percent of these centers are located in high schools, 33% in elementary schools, 16% in middle schools, and 13% in mixed schools. Only 9% of SBHCs are sponsored by the school system, 29% by hospitals, 22% by health departments, 18% by health centers, 24% by non-profit health organizations or a mix of institutions. New and growing resources are dental clinics now located in 1.7% SBHCs.

School-based health services are comprehensive, accessible, affordable, and culturally acceptable (Terwilliger, 1994). They have been associated with improved health outcomes, less absenteeism and fewer dropouts (Barnet, Arroyo, Devoe, & Duggan, 2004) and increased academic achievement (McCord, Klein, Foy, & Fothergill, 1993). The use of telehealth in SBHCs increases efficiency of services and reduces professional isolation (Young & Ireson, 2003). More research studies are needed to confirm these findings.

The National Assembly of School-Based Health Care (NASBHC), Center for Evaluation and Quality promotes an interdisciplinary research and evaluation agenda for SBHCs. Important research agendas have also been developed for school nursing services, rural education, and children's mental health. In 1994, 50 nongovernmental and governmental organizations came together to establish a research agenda for school nursing. By 1998, recommendations of this group included the importance of collaborations within schools and communities "who share the common cause of improving health and access to health care for the school-aged population" (Bradley, 1998, p. 20). In the Report of the Surgeon General's Conference on Children's Mental Health: A National Action Agenda, developed through a collaboration between the Department of Health and Human Services (DHHS), the Department of Education (DOE) and the Department of Justice, schools have an important role to play in proactive identification of mental health disorders in children and youth (US Public Health Service & Office of the Surgeon General, 2000). Finally, A McREL report describes a "limitless number of possibilities for a rural education research agenda" (Arnold, 2004, p. 1) with the following nine priority topics: "opportunity to learn, school size and student achievement, teacher quality, administrator quality, school and district capacity, school finance, local control and alternative organizational structures, school choice, and community and parent aspirations and expectations" (pp. 1–2).

Rural schools and rural communities have unique challenges in promoting the education and well-being of America's children. These challenges require further research and collaboration of many partners including students and families, educators and administrators, health care providers, and policy makers. Together, we can help children come to school healthy to learn while they learn to stay healthy.

## Structuring Rural School-Based Health Services for Success

Ideally, school-based health services are one component of a larger comprehensive approach to addressing needs of children and families. In a perfect world, this system of school-linked services takes the form of a newly developed system, as opposed to an added-on component. In helping this to occur, decisions about the following structural and organizational issues are key:

- Should services be school- or community-based?;
- What does collaboration among the different professionals and service systems that support school-linked services look like in practice?;
- What are the barriers and voices of opposition to school-linked services in rural communities?;

- Can confidentiality provisions be maintained without sacrificing collaboration?

## *School- versus Community-Based Services*

The term, school-linked services, refers to health and social service programs in affiliation with schools. Dryfoos (1994) asserts that the school has emerged as "the one piece of real estate in declining communities that is publicly owned, centrally located and consistently used, at least by children" (p. 139). This makes the school the most likely institution in the community to organize a comprehensive service delivery system for children and their families. Within this concept are two different models of operationalizing these services: school-based and community-based. When the Florida legislature adopted the label, "full-service school" they outlined these two models by calling for the creation of schools that integrate "education, medical, social and/or human services that are beneficial to meeting the needs of children and youth and their families on school grounds *or* [italics added] in locations which are easily accessible" (Dryfoos, 1994, p. 142).

Within these two models, of school and community-based, there are advocates, attributes and limitations to each. The major argument for school-based services is the access it provides, both between children and families and their services providers, as well as between providers and school personnel, for consultation and ongoing collaboration (Cervera, 1990; Harold & Harold, 1991; Larson, Gomby, Shiono, Lewit, & Behrman, 1992; Tyack, 1992). No other institution in the country has the legal mandate for access to children that the school holds. In addition, some cite an increase in attendance with school-based health services. For example, "if a child complains of a headache, the family may more likely send him/her to school because there is someone at the school" (Pires-Hestor, 1992, p. 9). This access to children is a natural bridge to their families and communities, yet the school grounds themselves are vastly underutilized. "With a few notable exceptions, schools are open for six hours on weekdays and closed tight all weekend and during vacations." "Tragically, this strategic real estate — so well-suited to meet family needs — remains vastly underused" (Murphy, 1993, p. 645).

Proponents of community-based services cite a number of arguments that counterbalance the advantages of access. One is the concern of institutional rigidity. When services are school-based it is easy for the school, as host, to take on the role of lead agency (Capper, 1994; Chaskin & Richman, 1993). Chaskin and Richman emphasize the difficulties that ensue when any organization, school or other, takes a lead role, and potentially molds services to fit "institutional requirements, priorities, and world view of the school" (p. 111). A second issue concerns the suitability of the school as a center for those families who associate the school with failure and difficulty. This is especially the case in rural areas where illiteracy rates are higher than in urban areas (Caudill, 1993) and where the school is associated with discomfort as opposed to being a haven. Might rural families with negative associations with the school be more likely to utilize services provided by non-school entities? Additionally there are concerns about adequacy of professionals trained as educators in taking on the role of service provider. Perhaps this role is best left to those trained in, and employed by agencies dedicated to health and human service delivery. Often this division of labor is supported by the school, which is then left to focus on their mandate — teaching children. Lastly, in the absence of a model of true collaboration and shared leadership, many argue that a broader spectrum of services can develop when a *non*-school, i.e., health care agency takes on the leadership role, maintaining its own fiscal and other responsibility for service provision. Some argue that this type of arrangement supports the widest breadth of service. The issue of breadth is critical, as numerous types of important services and populations can be left out when services are on school grounds. The services which often have opposition to their placement on school grounds include pregnancy prevention, substance abuse treatment, and mental health services. Populations left out include pregnant or ill students, temporarily being schooled elsewhere. In addition, community-based services operate year round, and are not restricted to a school's academic calendar (Dryfoos, 1994).

When proponents of school-based health services develop programs, they need to pay attention to the arguments for community-based services, and attempt to create programs that are not bound by the potential limitations. Those collaborating may need to assess the school they are organizing around, to see whether or not the argument for access is outweighed by the concerns about institutional rigidity, families' prior feelings about the school and the degree of freedom in service provision.

## *Collaboration in Practice*

While the ideal school-based health program is embedded in a larger network of integrated services, this is not easy to accomplish. The true meaning of a community-led system of school-linked services does not refer to a school or to a health or social service system as leader, but to a collaboration among providers, including schools, health and mental health centers, parks, libraries, and other significant community institutions, responding together to the needs of its resident families (Chaskin & Richman, 1993). Unfortunately, disciplines and agencies often defend their turf and thus, the ideal of collaboration is not so easy to implement. Dryfoos (1994) suggests the following definition for collaboration that often best characterizes it in practice: "an unnatural act between nonconsenting adults" (p. 149).

Melaville and colleagues (Melaville & Blank, 1991; Melaville, Blank, & Asayes, 1993) outline concrete conditions and processes that support the building of a collaborative model of comprehensive services for children and families, directly applicable to the development of school-linked services. They cite the major challenge of developing "a process of working together that is flexible enough to allow adjustments to new circumstances, while staying focused on long-term goals" (Melaville et al., 1993, p. 19). The first stage in their five stage process for change involves the coming together of a small group of committed people. These participants begin to identify and include key stakeholders, make a commitment to collaborate, and establish a unifying theme. They set precedents for shared leadership, ground rules for working together, and discuss financing their initial planning efforts. In the second stage, partners create a shared vision of how they would like a comprehensive service delivery system to look, develop a mission statement and a set of goals to set them on their way. In the third stage, members begin to focus on specifics. They define their geographic area and design a "prototype delivery system" (p. 53). They develop technical tools and interagency agreements to support their efforts. These often take the form of case management structures and mechanisms to guide issues of confidentiality. Caudill (1993) identifies case management as a critical function to support service utilization in rural counties. This refinement and specification of a plan often leads to the addition of new partners to the collaborative effort. In the fourth stage, partners begin to implement the prototype. This provides feedback that in turn guides policy and practices of the participating organizations. This is often the time that an evaluation system is designed and implemented. In the fifth and last stage, the prototype is expanded to the desired scale, for a system of integrated services. This stage often includes building the community constituency, a governance structure, a long-range fiscal strategy, and inter-professional training (Melaville et al., 1993).

Melaville and Blank (1991) outline five critical variables necessary to support collaboration. The first is the external environment, including the neighborhood's social and political climate. The best external environment for establishing school-linked services would be one where key decision makers value this effort, and support relationships among potential partners. The second important variable in creating and sustaining collaborative efforts is an effective system of communication and problem-solving, which emerges from a shared vision. The focus needs to remain on the establishment of effective services, the opportunity for learning, and the hope of building a system greater than the sum of its parts, as opposed to what is lost in sharing power and compromising.

The third variable, people, addresses the importance of leadership from within the collaborative: (a) the inclusion of key players in the community, and (b) the critical role of staff in moving from vision to service delivery. As a broad reaching community initiative, efforts towards collaborative school-linked services require representation that reflects the community including school personnel, service providers, parents, and other key community players. Support from high level school officials, including school board members, superintendent and principal are critical to have behind the project. They influence important issues like resources and space. Many experts document the importance of ongoing parental involvement in school-linked services efforts. Parental involvement assures utilization of services, and a whole host of cognitive, affective and behavioral outcome measures that school-linked services look towards (Chavkin & Brown, 1992; Comer, 1988; Constable, 1992; Dryfoos, 1994; Rosenthal, 1995). Parental involvement runs the gamut from involvement in hiring and firing decisions to representation on committees. True collaboration is more likely to occur the more there is equal representation in planning and service delivery from families, school and health, and social service personnel (Bronstein, 2003; Shedlin, 1990). Dryfoos (1994) notes that elementary school parents are easier to involve, simply because it is a time when parents need to be closer and more involved than they do when their children reach high school. Issues of confidentiality also arise in service programs with older adolescents, where service providers are not bound to share information with parents, and on the contrary, are sometimes legally bound not to share. Another important, but often overlooked participant group is children, those who are most dramatically affected by the new programming. By including children in the planning and implementation, a program is more likely to reflect their needs and desires. It also gives them genuine responsibility for what happens in their school community and provides them with opportunities to develop leadership skills (Children's Aid Society, 1993).

The fourth variable critical in supporting school-linked services concerns the policies that guide institutions, and the degree to which these disparate rules and regulations can be made to complement each other. There is a natural tendency for participants to "maintain their distinctive organizational characteristics" (Melaville & Blank, 1991, p. 29). This gives rise to the commonly cited "turf issues," which Dryfoos (1994) describes as "having your mother-in-law come and stay in your house" (p. 154). These differences take the form of disagreements among professionals from different disciplines, agency guidelines, and at times, legal statutes. In school-linked services a legal issue might arise from services attempting to reach students who have dropped out of school, when the school no longer receives funding to support these students who are not enrolled.

The fifth condition Melaville and Blank (1991) discuss is resources. Ways the availability of resources impacts school-linked services includes: "whether or not the changes in services and service delivery that the joint effort has established will become permanently institutionalized and the size of the population that will eventually benefit from these changes" (p. 31).

## Barriers and Opposition

Those voicing opposition to school-linked services claim a range of concerns. These include the fear that schools will offer too many diverse services and not enough substance, the fear of "inflicting help" on those who don't want it, concern about schools getting into issues that are "personal" in nature and perhaps the largest and loudest objection to schools as "sex clinics" (Dryfoos, 1994; Pacheco, Powell, & Cole, 1991). These concerns may become especially apparent in rural communities where more traditional values prevail and where there is a strong ethos that families take care of their own (Caudill, 1993). In addition to these articulated objections, come the obstacles that inherently arise when diverse agencies attempt to build a new collaborative. These include: (a) institutional disincentives; (b) historical and ideological barriers; (c) power disparities among stakeholders; (d) societal-level dynamics, including the trend toward individualism in this country, differing perceptions of the level of acceptable risk, added technical complexity and established political and institutional norms (Gray, 1995). In order to combat these obstacles, partners must consistently attend to them through broad-scale participation in, and communication of, each stage in the development and implementation of school-linked services. The fact that these services are so dependent on such a range of levels of support, i.e., their surrounding neighborhoods for participation, their community structure which influences the demographics and problems confronting the local residents, the states for policy, law and funding makes the challenge of broad-scale participation and communication only possible to exist as an ideal. Yet the closer one gets to this ideal, the more likely it is that a true collaborative can develop, and that system change can occur. It is the enormity of the relevant actors and factors in this work that encouraged Bartelt (1995) to talk about the "macro-ecology of educational outcomes."

## Confidentiality

The existence of confidentiality provisions can support or deter inter-agency collaborative relationships. Families feel safe and respected when they know their rights to privacy are protected and are more apt to engage with services where this is the case. At the same time, professionals view the limits on the flow of information and potentially on the delivery of services imposed by confidentiality regulations as major impediments to collaboration.

While it is easy to become frustrated with confidentiality provisions, it is important to be aware of the variety of ways they support the privacy of children and families. A continuing education program produced by the Center for Mental Health in schools (n.d.) draws from the work of Soler and Peters from the early 1990s "The reasons for respecting privacy of children and families include the following:... protect embarrassing personal information from disclosure... prevent improper dissemination of information about children and families that might increase the likelihood of discrimination or harm against them... protect personal security... family security... job security... avoid prejudice or differential treatment... encourage individuals to make use of services designed to help them" (p. II–72). On the other side of this issue are equally valid rationales in support of sharing information. These include: (a) conducting comprehensive assessments; (b) providing all necessary services; (c) avoiding duplication and encouraging efficiency; (d) encouraging coordinated and continuous service plans; (e) facilitating the monitoring of services; (f) helping to make services more family-focused; (g) serving the needs of the broader community; and (h) promoting public safety (Greenberg & Levy, 1992). Confidentiality provisions come from a variety of state and federal sources as well as professional and ethical standards. It is critical to understand which provisions govern information sharing in each particular agency, and for which clients. The focus needs to be broader than a look at whether or not information can be shared. Instead the focus should reflect a look at ways to meet legitimate service goals within what is possible under the law. The foundation of sharing information that is otherwise protected by confidentiality provisions, is through "informed consent." This means that consent "must be given voluntarily and must be 'informed' — that is, the individual must understand fully what information will be exchanged, with whom it will be shared and how it will be used. Consent must be documented in writing, usually on a signed release form" (Greenberg & Levy, 1992, p. 13). When a person is not old enough for a consent to be legally binding, a parent or guardian may sign. Despite this, several collaborators request children's signatures as a way to encourage their involvement and sense of ownership over their participation in the services being provided. Some state statutes allow minors to consent to the release of information regarding health issues such as sexually transmitted diseases, pregnancy, rape, or substance use. In addition, some states have either court recognized "mature" or emancipated minors who may provide consent in their own health care and release of information; or the health care of their children, if they are parents. Sometimes immigrants are fearful of signing releases, concerned that information shared may put them at risk of deportation. This fear can be ameliorated by clearly stating on the release form that no personal information will be given to the Immigration and Naturalization Service (Greenberg & Levy, 1992; Soler & Peters, 1993).

While confidentiality is an issue to address in all agency work, it is critical in school-linked services where the best collaboratives are often the most far reaching, and where issues of information sharing are frequent and complex. Greenberg and Levy (1992) recommend that information sharing not be among the first tasks tackled as a collaborative is developed. They argue that it is critical to have strong working relationships and commitment to the collaborative prior to addressing the sharing of information. Holding off on this issue allows a basis of trust to develop. They do, however, advocate that participants clearly put this issue on the future agenda as a way of asserting that it is important, will not be ignored, and will be addressed after other aspects of planning for joint action. Like the other issues discussed — pros and cons for school- vs. community-based programs, how to actualize collaboration in practice, and awareness of the barriers and opposition to school-linked services, confidentiality, when handled thoughtfully, can add, rather than take away from collaborative efforts to build and sustain school-linked services.

## Case Study

The following case study provides an example of the type of educational, health, and social struggles children experience in rural schools. The collaboration of many partners is necessary to make a difference.

## *My Tooth Hurts*

On a typical day, in a rural school, five-year-old "Peggy" was so uncomfortable that she could not eat her lunch. Her teacher brought Peggy to the school-based health center at lunchtime complaining, "My tooth hurts!" A physical exam of Peggy's mouth revealed hot, swollen gum tissue surrounding one decayed tooth. After the exam, the center's nurse practitioner suspected that the little girl had a dental abscess caused by severe cavities.

The center immediately contacted Peggy's mother by phone. Peggy's mom had no insurance and — although she had looked for one — she had been unable to find a dentist who would care for her daughter. She quickly gave permission for the center staff to give Peggy a pain reliever every day so that she could at least eat her lunch.

That same day, Peggy was sent home with a prescription for an antibiotic to temporarily treat her abscessed tooth. In addition to helping Peggy feel better, the nurse practitioner referred her mother to the center's social worker to begin addressing the problem of getting her daughter access to care.

Fortunately, the social worker determined that Peggy was eligible for a subsidized Child Health Insurance Program. In addition, the center found a pediatric dentist in a nearby state who was willing to accept Peggy as a patient. To ease the financial burden on Peggy's mother, the social worker helped arrange transportation needed to get Peggy to the dentist. At the dentist's office, Peggy had the abscess treated, some teeth pulled, and still others restored. After a long period of severe dental problems, this young patient was ready to focus on enjoying school and learning again, without pain. (Terwilliger, 1997)

## REFERENCES

Arnold, M. (2004). *Guiding rural schools and districts: A research agenda.* Aurora, CO: Mid-continent Research for Education and Learning.

Barnet, B., Arroyo, C., Devoe, M., & Duggan, A. K. (2004). Reduced school dropout rates among adolescent mothers receiving school-based prenatal care. *Archives of Pediatrics & Adolescent Medicine, 158*(3), 262–268.

Bartelt, D. W. (1995). The macroecology of educational outcomes. In L. C. Rigsby, M. C. Reynolds & M. C. Wang (Eds.), *School-community connections*: Exploring issues for research and practice (pp. 159–192). San Francisco: Jossey-Bass.

Bradley, B. J. (1998). Establishing a research agenda for school nursing. *Journal of School Health, 68*(2), 53–61.

Bronstein, L. R. (2003). A model for interdisciplinary collaboration. *Social Work, 48*(3), 297–306.

Capper, C. A. (1994). "We're not housed in an institution, we're housed in the community": possibilities and consequences of neighborhood-based interagency collaboration. *Educational Administration Quarterly, 30,* 257–277.

Caudill, M. H. (1993). School social work services in rural appalachian systems: identifying and closing the gaps. *Social Work in Education, 15,* 179–185.

CDC, & Coordinating Center for Health Promotion. (2007). Healthy youth! An investment in our nation's future 2007. Retrieved March 3, 2007 from http://www.cdc.gov/healthyyouth/about/pdf/HealthyYouth.2007.pdf

CDC, & Health Resources and Services Administration. (2004). Healthy people 2010: Educational and community-based programs. Retrieved October 13, 2004 from http://www.healthypeople.gov/Document/HTML/Volume1/07Ed.htm

Center for Health and Health Care in Schools. (2004). Critical caring on the front line. George Washington University School of Public Health and Health Services. Washington, DC. Retrieved October 13, 2004, from http://www.healthinschools.org/FS/fsmap.html

Center for Mental Health in Schools at UCLA (nd). *Addressing barriers to learning: New directions for mental health in schools.* Los Angeles, CA: School Mental Health Project, Dept. of Psychology, UCLA. Retrieved October 13, 2004 from http://smhp.psych.ucla.edu/specres.htm#guidebooks

Cervera, N. (1990). Community agencies in schools: Interlopers or colleagues? *Social Work in Education, 12*(2), 118–133.

Chaskin, R. J., & Richman, H. A. (1993). Concerns about school-linked services: Institution-based versus community-based models. *Education and Urban Society, 25,* 205–211.

Chavkin, N. F., & Brown, K. (1992). School social workers building a multiethnic family-school-community partnership. Coalition for PRIDE (Positive, Responsible Individuals Desiring an Education) in San Marcos Consolidated Independent School District. *Social Work in Education, 14*(3), 160–164.

Children's Aid Society. (1993). *Building a community school: A revolutionary design in public schools.* New York: Author.

Comer, J. P. (1988). Educating poor minority children. *Scientific American, 259*(5), 42–48.

Constable, R. T. (1992). The new school reform and the school social worker. *Social Work in Education, 14*(2), 106–113.

Dryfoos, J. G. (1994). *Full-service schools: A revolution in health and social services for children, youth, and families.* San Francisco, CA: Jossey-Bass.

Fisher, C., Hunt, P., Kann, L., Kolbe, L., Patterson, B., & Wechsler, H. (2003). Building a healthier future through school health programs. In *Promising practices in chronic disease prevention and control: A public health framework for action* (pp. 9-2–9-25). Atlanta, GA: Department of Health and Human Services, CDC.

Gamm, L., Hutchison, L. L., Dabney, B. J., & Dorsey, A. M. (2003a). *Rural healthy people 2010: A companion document to healthy people 2010 (Vol. 1).* College Station, TX: Texas A&M University System Health Science Center, School of Rural Public Health, Southwest Rural Health Research Center.

Gamm, L., Hutchison, L. L., Dabney, B. J., & Dorsey, A. M. (2003b). *Rural healthy people 2010: A companion document to healthy people 2010 (Vol. 2).* College Station, TX: Texas A&M University System Health Science Center, School of Rural Public Health, Southwest Rural Health Research Center.

Gray, B. (1995). Obstacles to success in educational collaborations. In L. C. Rigsby, M. C. Reynolds & M. C. Wang (Eds.), *School-community connections: Exploring issues for research and practice* (pp. 71–100). San Francisco: Jossey-Bass.

Green-Hernandez, C. (1992). Being there and caring: A philosophical analysis and theoretical model of professional nurse caring in rural environments. In P. Winstead-Fry, T. J. Churchill & R. V. Shippee-Rice (Eds.), *Rural health nursing: Stories of creativity, commitment, and connectedness* (pp. 31–54). New York: National League for Nursing.

Greenberg, M., & Levy, J. (1992). *Confidentiality and collaboration: Information sharing in interagency efforts.* Denver, CO: Education Commission of the States.

Harold, N. B., & Harold, R. D. (1991). School-based clinics: A vehicle for social work intervention. *Social Work in Education, 13*(3), 185–194.

Ihlenfeld, J. (2004). Community-oriented nurse in the schools. In M. Stanhope & J. Lancaster (Eds.), *Community & public health nursing* (6th ed., pp. 1042–1065). St. Louis, MO: Mosby.

Krause, C., O'Sullivan, A., Terwilliger, S., & Nierstedt, N. (2004). *Anticipatory guidance for positive youth development in adolescence.* Retrieved October 15, 2004, from http://www.nursingworld.org/mods/mod620/ceythtoc.htm

Larson, C. S., Gomby, D. S., Shiono, P. H., Lewit, E. M., & Behrman, R. E. (1992). School-linked services: Analysis. *Future of Children, 2*(1), 6–18.

Long, K. A., & Weinert, C. (1992). Rural nursing: developing the theory base. In P. Winstead-Fry, T. J. Churchill & R. V. Shippee-Rice (Eds.), *Rural health nursing: Stories of creativity, commitment, and connectedness* (pp. 389–406). New York: National League for Nursing.

McCord, M. T., Klein, J. D., Foy, J. M., & Fothergill, K. (1993). School-based clinic use and school performance. *Journal of Adolescent Health, 14*(2), 91–98.

Melaville, A. I., & Blank, M. J. (1991). *What it takes: Structuring interagency partnerships to connect children and families with comprehensive services.* Washington, DC: Education and Human Services Consortium.

Melaville, A. I., Blank, M. J., & Asayes, G. (1993). *Together we can: A guide for crafting a profamily system of education and human services.* Washington, DC: U.S. Dept. of Education Office of Educational Research and Improvement U.S. Dept. of Health and Human Services Office of the Assistant Secretary for Planning and Evaluation

Murphy, J. A. (1993). What's in? What's out? American education in the nineties. *Phi Delta Kappan, 74,* 641–646.

Pacheco, M., Powell, W., & Cole, C. (1991). School-based clinics: The politics of change. *Journal of School Health, 61,* 92–94.

Pastore, D. R., & Techow, B. (2004). Adolescent school-based health care: A description of two sites in their 20th year of service. *The Mount Sinai Journal of Medicine, 71*(3), 191–196.

Pires-Hestor, L. (1992). *School-based health clinics in an "education" society.* Paper presented at the Third Annual Conference on Universities, Community Schools, and Job Training. Philadelphia, PA.

Ricketts, T. C. (Ed.). (1999). *Rural Health in the United States.* New York: Oxford University Press.

Rosenthal, B. S. (1995). The influence of social support on school completion among Haitians. *Social Work in Education, 17*(1), 30–39.

Rural Assistance Center. (2004). *Schools information guide.* Retrieved October 13, 2004, from http://www.raconline.org/info_guides/schools

Shedlin, A., Jr. (1990). Shelter from the storm. The school as the center of social services for children. *The American School Board Journal, 177,* 12–16.

Soler, M., & Peters, C. (1993). *Who should know what? Confidentiality and information sharing in service integration.* Des Moines, IA: National Center for Service Integration.

Terwilliger, S. (1997). My tooth hurts. In C. A. Shearer (Ed.), *Success stories: How school-based health centers make a difference* (p. 2). Washington, DC: National Health and Education Consortium.

Terwilliger, S. H. (1994). Early access to health care services through a rural school-based health center. *Journal of School Health, 64*(7), 284–289.

Tyack, D. (1992). Health and social services in public schools: Historical perspectives. *Future of Children, 2*(1), 19–31.

U.S. Public Health Service, & Office of the Surgeon General. (2000). *Report of the Surgeon General's conference on children's mental health: A national action agenda.* Washington, DC: DHHS. retrieved from http://www.surgeongeneral.gov/topics/cmh/childreport.htm

Winstead-Fry, P. (1992). Family theory for rural research and practice. In P. Winstead-Fry, T. J. Churchill & R. V. Shippee-Rice (Eds.), *Rural health nursing: Stories of creativity, commitment, and connectedness* (pp. 127–148). New York: National League for Nursing.

Young, T. L., & Ireson, C. (2003). Effectiveness of school-based telehealth care in urban and rural elementary schools. *Pediatrics, 112*(5), 1088–1094.

*Chapter 3*

# A Community Action Mandate for Oral Health in Rural Populations

SARAH HALL GUELDNER, CAROLYN PIERCE,
PETER BEATTY, FREDERICK J. LACEY, LYNNE B. LACEY,
LEANN LESPERANCE, JOYCE HYATT,
FRAN SRNKA-DEBNAR, SUSAN TERWILLIGER,
AND LUCY BIANCO

**Abstract:** The purpose of this paper is to bring attention to the almost silent epidemic of poor oral health that is gripping our country, and to examine in particular the oral health needs of persons who live in remote areas. Implications of poor oral health are highlighted, with particular emphasis on the serious impact of poor oral health on general health status. Barriers to adequate care are discussed, including reimbursement issues and inaccessibility, especially for persons who live in remote areas and may not have transportation to travel for care. The low priority generally assigned to oral health will also be discussed. Finally, the authors put forward a "call to action" for addressing the problem. Community models based within a multidisciplinary approach are offered for consideration.

## The State of Oral Health Care in the United States

The 2000 Surgeon General's Report addressed the epidemic of oral disease that "is affecting our most vulnerable citizens — poor children, the elderly, and many members of racial and ethnic minority groups" (U.S. Department of Health and Human Services [USDHHS], 2000, p. 1). Employed adults living in the United States (U.S.) lose more than 164 million hours of work each year due to oral health problems (USDHHS, 2000, p. 3). Less than two-thirds or about 66% of adults report having visited a dentist in the past year. Those with incomes at or above the poverty level are twice as likely to report a dental visit in the past 12 months as those who are below the poverty level (p. 3). "Customer service industry employees lose 2–4 times more work hours than executives or professional workers" (National Center for Chronic Disease Prevention and Health Promotion [NCCDPHP], 2006a, p. 1). These statistics confirm (USDHHS, 2000) the impact of poor oral health on the fiber of our country; a problem that often gets worse as individuals retire from the workforce and lose their dental insurance, at an age when they are most likely to need care.

Life expectancy in the U.S. has increased from 47 years in 1900 to nearly 77 years in 2000 (p. 276), and persons who reach 65 years of age have a high probability of living to age 80 (USDHHS, 2000b). Since persons 55 years and older are the major consumers of health care (Janes et al., 1999) the dramatic increase in this segment of the population is imposing heavy demands on the oral health care system, which is already strained by a severe shortage of dental providers and services. With the introduction of fluoride into community water systems in the mid-1940s, more people are retaining their natural dentition into advanced age, but large dental restorations and other oral problems need continuing care. Plaque also builds up faster on older teeth, partly because of decreasing ability to maintain proper oral hygiene and partly due to decreased salivary flow. Consequently, the most severe oral problems are found in the oldest and sickest patients. It is also important to note that while community water fluoridation is the most effective measure of improving oral health (Centers for Disease Control and Prevention [CDC], 2001), more than one half of the U.S. population, mostly rural dwellers, do not have access to this community resource. In 2000, only 26 states and the District of Columbia had achieved the Health Policy 2010 goal of providing access to fluoridated public water supplies to 75% of their population (CDC, 2001). This places rural communities at greatest risk, since most rural families have their own wells and would not have the benefit of public fluoridation.

At least half of the non-institutionalized people over age 55 have periodontitis, sometimes referred to as gum disease, and severe periodontitis affects 23% of adults who are 65–74 years of age (NCCDPHP, 2006b; USDHHS, 2000). Men tend to have more serious disease than women, and people at the lowest socioeconomic level have the most severe periodontal disease (USDHHS, 2000, p. 3). One out of four people age 65 and older have lost all of their teeth (NCCDPHP, 2006b). Since older people did not grow up in a time when oral care was a priority, they may not have developed the regular dental habits that now are recommended i.e., brushing twice daily, using dental floss, and regular dental checkups, and may not be as aware of their oral care needs. Most cannot afford optimum dental care, and many are embarrassed about their teeth, particularly if they feel they have not taken good care of them. The high prevalence of multi-medication therapies in older persons may further impact oral health in elders, and institutionalized elders are at great risk for poor oral health (Ebersole, Hess, & Luggen, 2003; Hobbins, 1999).

Oral and pharyngeal cancers are diagnosed in over 30,000 Americans each year, primarily in the elderly (NCCDPHP, 2006b). The prognosis is poor, often due to delayed diagnosis, resulting in 7,400 deaths each year. The five-year survival rate for white patients is 56%, whereas only 34% of African American patients survive (p. 2). Every year more than 400,000 cancer patients undergoing chemotherapy suffer from painful mouth ulcers and dry mouth from reduced salivary flow (USDHHS, 2000). Patients with weakened immune systems, such as those with HIV or organ transplant, are at higher risk for oral problems. There is also growing evidence that bacteria from decayed teeth and periodontal tissues may travel via the bloodstream to other parts of the body, contributing to the incidence of heart attack, stroke, diabetes, premature births, and infection at the site of joint replacements (Petersen & Yamamoto, 2005; USDHHS, 2000).

## *Disparities in Oral Health Care*

The Surgeon General also described the profound oral health disparities within the American population that must be addressed (USDHHS, 2000). Minority segments of the population are at higher risk for less than optimal care. One-third of white Americans, nearly half of Hispanics (47%) and African Americans (43%), and two-thirds (66%) of our American Indians/Alaskan Natives did not receive dental services in 2001 (NCCDPHP, 2002, p. 2). Poverty creates the greatest disparity; those with incomes at or above the poverty level are twice as likely to visit a dentist as those with lower incomes. Oral health needs are particularly urgent in underserved rural states (Beetstra et al., 2002; Krause, Mosca, & Livingston, 2003). Rural adults are less likely than their urban counterparts to be able to pay for dental care, and are less likely to report dental visits in the past year. Further, a higher proportion of rural residents than urban residents are edentulous and report poor dental status (Beetstra et al., 2002; Vargus, Yellowitz, & Hayes, 2003). Persons in rural areas may be self employed or not be able to get off from work and often encounter serious transportation problems; so they tend to let their dental problems go and seek emergency dental treatment only when the pain becomes unbearable (Heaton, Smith, & Raybould, 2004). For these and other reasons, providing oral health care to rural population presents a major challenge (Mouradian et al., 2003). Lack of community water fluoridation, dental workforce shortages, cost of care, and geographical barriers all aggravate oral health and access problems in rural areas. Inequities in access to oral health care especially affect low-income individuals living in underserved areas. Children and elders from low-income and minority families and those with special needs are at particular risk. It is estimated that as many as 11% of our nation's rural population have never received dental treatment (Krause et al., 2003).

## *Children*

Dental caries, tooth decay, is the single most common chronic childhood disease; it is five times more common than asthma and seven times more common than hay fever (Gonsalves, Skelton, Smith, Hardison, & Ferretti, 2004, p. 544). Eighteen percent of children aged two to four have had dental caries, and the average number of decayed, missing, and filled teeth among children aged two to four years has remained unchanged over the past 25 years. More than 50 percent of five- to nine-year-old children have at least one decayed, missing, or filled tooth, and that proportion increases to 78 percent among 17-year-olds (Mouradian, Wehr, & Crall, 2000; USDHHS, 2000, p. 63). Poor children suffer twice as many dental caries as their more affluent peers, and their disease is more likely to be untreated. The differences between poor and non-poor children continue into adolescence. One out of four children in America is born into poverty, and children living below the poverty line, annual income of $17,000 for a family of four, have more severe and untreated decay

(Mouradian et al., 2000; USDHHS, 2000, p. 63). One-fourth (25%) of poor children have not seen a dentist before entering kindergarten. The Surgeon General (USDHHS, 2000, p. 7) emphasized that getting off to a healthy start is crucial to life long oral health, and these statistics show that we are nowhere near that goal. More than 51 million school hours are lost each year to dental-related illness (p. 2). Poor children suffer nearly 12 times more restricted activity days than children from higher income families (p. 2).

Ability to pay is a strong predictor of access to dental care (Allender & Spradley, 2001). "Uninsured children are 2.5 times less likely than insured children to receive dental care. Children from families without dental insurance are three times more likely to have dental needs than children with either public or private insurance" (USDHHS, 2000, p. 2). Medicaid has not been able to fill the gap in providing dental care to poor children (Mouradian et al., 2000). In a year-long study, less than one in five Medicaid-covered children received a single dental visit. For each child without Medicaid insurance, there are at least 2.6 children without dental insurance. Even the Children's Health Insurance Program (CHIP) will not be able to close this gap (USDHHS, 2000, p. 8).

## *Clinical Implications*

Many factors have been identified that increase a person's risk for poor oral health (see Table 1). It is important that health care providers from across disciplines assess their clients regularly for these factors. Selected clinical issues will be discussed in the paragraphs below.

### *Prevention and Treatment*

Meticulous oral hygiene and avoidance of risk factors when possible are keys in the quest for prevention of oral disease, and can only be achieved by educating the public as well as all healthcare providers about their importance. Persons who wear dentures should also be included in this educational program, since they are also at higher risk for oral disease. Once oral pathology is present, treatment demands the attention of dental professionals. Therefore, it is important to teach the public and non-dental professionals how to recognize signs of oral pathology so that they can help persons to access treatment. It is also imperative that formal or informal caregivers provide daily oral hygiene for impaired elders, young children, and others who are unable to perform these activities independently.

**Table 1**
*Risk Factors for Edentulism, Caries, and Gum Disease*

| Lack of knowledge related to dental care | Poor oral hygiene |
|---|---|
| Low socioeconomic status | Lack of access to dental services |
| Lack of dental insurance | Advanced age |
| Racial or ethnic minority status | Less than a high school education or low levels of parental education |
| Poor dietary habits | Poor general health status |
| Some types of medication and medical treatments | Smoking |
| Excessive use of alcohol | Insufficient exposure to fluoride |
| History of high caries in older siblings | Reduced salivary flow |
| Use of orthodontic appliances | Diabetes, cancer, AIDS, or osteoporosis |

(USDHHS, 2000)

## *Management of Dry Mouth*

Certain medical conditions and medications cause dry mouth, leaving the mouth without enough saliva to wash away food and neutralize plaque. People with dry mouth are more susceptible to tooth decay and periodontal disease (National Institute of Dental and Craniofacial Research [NIDCR], 2006). Over 400 commonly used medications may produce dry mouth, including antihistamines, diuretics, pain relievers, antihypertensives and antidepressants (NCCDPHP, 2006b, p. 2; USDHHS, 2000). Individuals in long term care facilities, about 5% of the elderly, are at higher risk, since they take an average of eight drugs each day (USDHHS, 2000, p. 3). Sugarless gum, oral rinses, or artificial saliva products may offer some relief for this problem. Meticulous oral hygiene is imperative for these individuals.

## Nutritional Aspects

Effective mastication is critical to good nutrition, and intervention is required when the ability to chew is altered by oral pathology. People with dentures, loose or missing teeth, or painful gum disease often place themselves on a self-imposed restrictive diet of soft foods, since biting into fresh fruits and vegetables or meat is difficult and painful. Thus they are at substantial risk for developing malnutrition. Optimum oral health allows a choice of more nutritious food, as well as a more pleasant eating experience. The opposite situation is also true; malnutrition, especially with a prolonged deficit in calcium and protein intake, may lead to increased dental problems. Positive nutrition helps prevent, while poor eating habits can promote caries. For instance, eating fiber rich fruits and vegetables stimulates salivary flow, which in turn helps prevent tooth decay. On the other hand, the frequent consumption of refined carbohydrates in snack foods contributes to the formation of dental caries and demineralization. Compelling evidence of the importance of oral health to well being is found in a recent nutritional study of 386 community dwelling persons which showed that eating problems were significantly correlated with hospitalization (Jensen, Friedmann, Coleman, & Smiciklas-Wright, 2001).

## Oral Care for Elders in Long Term Care

Residents of long term care facilities are at particular risk for poor oral heath. In a study conducted by a team of Swedish nurses (Wardh, Hallberg, Berggren, Andersson, & Sorensen, 2000), virtually all long term care nursing staff and other health care providers rated oral care as important; but when faced with work day realities, other activities were almost always given higher priority, at the expense of oral care. Other authors have reported similar findings (Vargas, Kramarow, & Yellowitz, 2001). A more subtle indication that oral care is not considered a part of general nursing care is the noticeable absence of specific routines for assisting with oral care, and its omission from care plans except when there is a serious problem. Reports also reveal that it is unclear to staff whose responsibility it is to provide oral care. As a result, most staff assume that someone else, a family member or staff on another shift, is doing it (Wardh et al.,

2000). Virtually all of the staff interviewed by Wardh and colleagues (2000) felt that assisting residents with oral hygiene was burdensome, and several described it as "repulsive" or "disgusting." One nursing assistant commented on how difficult it is to gain access to the oral cavity against resistance. Another was afraid of being bitten by a demented or confused patient who perhaps would not understand what was being done. In this regard, Hobbins (1999) noted that older adults with cognitive impairment are at special risk for inadequate oral care, and recommended that they be scheduled for comprehensive oral assessment as soon as possible after the onset of their cognitive decline, while they may still be able to understand instructions and cooperate to some degree with dental staff. Several authors have pointed out that nursing staff often have had minimal education in oral health, perhaps making it more likely that daily mouth care would be neglected when confronted with busy or troublesome circumstances. It is encouraging to note that guidelines for oral care for residents in long term care facilities are being developed (Fitzpatrick, 2000; Roberts, 2000).

Dental services available to residents of skilled nursing facilities are limited in regard to the time each resident is able to spend with the dentist. One of the *Healthy People 2010* objectives is to increase the proportion of long-term care residents who use the oral health care system each year. Data from 1997 indicate that only 19% of all nursing home residents received dental care in the previous year (NCCDPHP, 2001). Fortunately, New York State now requires that all long term care residents have an initial and yearly oral evaluations by a dentist or dental hygienist (New York State Department of Health, 1992).

## *Policy Implications*

The Surgeon General's office has affirmed oral health as integral to the general health and well-being of all Americans, and has mandated that it be included in the provision of health care and design of community programs (USDHHS, 2000). Likewise, the Academy of General Dentistry and the American Dental Association are committed to increasing the oral health literacy of health care professionals, policymakers, and the public, and encourages dentists to become more involved in community efforts to increase access to care for underserved populations.

## Barriers to Oral Care

Regular dental visits allow dental health professionals to provide preventive services and early diagnosis. Thus annual oral examinations are recommended for all children and adults, but are essential for the poorest and frailest of our society. In addition, people need ready access to emergency care for oral health problems. Unfortunately, significant barriers to adequate oral care exist.

### Shortage of Dental Professionals

Notable among the factors limiting access to oral care is the marked shortage of dental providers and services, particularly in underserved rural areas. According to the Health Resources and Services Administration, there are nearly 2000 Dental Health Professional Shortage Areas in non-metropolitan and frontier areas of the U.S. These areas are estimated to contain an underserved population of more than 14.7 million people and a need for up to 8000 additional dental practitioners to cover the total dental health professions service areas where over 40 million people currently live (USDHHS, 2005).

### Cost

The literature suggests that cost associated with oral care is the greatest barrier to access (Krause et al., 2003). Lack of dental insurance and inadequate reimbursement programs constitute major barriers to access to dental care in low-income segments of the population. "Most employers of low-wage workers do not offer a dental insurance benefit, ... if offered, the employee portion of the premium is not affordable for those earning less than 200% of the federal poverty level" (Beetstra et al., 2002, p. 1). In addition, persons who live in remote areas often are not employed by a company that offers dental insurance.

Dental insurance coverage is a strong correlate of dental care use, particularly among older adults. But because dental insurance is usually provided as an employer benefit, retired persons living in the U.S. are less likely to have dental insurance (Vargas et al., 2001, p. 6). "The situation may be worse for older women, who generally have lower incomes and may never have had dental insurance" (USDHHS, 2000, p. 3). Since many older adults are on a fixed income, lack of dental insurance and the rising cost of prescription drugs may cause them to forego preventative dental treatments (USDHHS, 2000).

Since 1960, more than 93% of dental care has been financed either as out-of-pocket paid directly to the dentist or through employment-based dental insurance benefits (USDHHS, 2000, p. 229). Although insurance coverage for dental care is increasing, it still lags behind medical insurance (p. 8). "For every child less under 18 years of age without medical insurance, there are at least two without dental insurance. For every adult 18 years or older without medical insurance, there are three without dental insurance" (p. 9). As a result an estimated 79% of dental services are paid directly by individuals. Medicaid funds dental care for the low-income and disabled elderly in some states, but reimbursements are below usual and customary fees (p. 3). Therefore, because of low reimbursement rates and the high administrative overhead needed to handle billing, most dentists, 75%, have chosen not to participate in the Medicaid Dental Program in the past. In fact, in 2002 only one percent of the Division of Medicaid expenditures were spent on dental services, and only 18.8 percent of children eligible for Medicaid received oral preventive services by dentists (USDHHS, 2000).

## *Transportation Challenges*

Transportation to and from oral health providers also may pose a significant problem for persons who live in geographically remote areas. Many older adults living in rural communities must depend on family and friends for transportation to a dental clinic. Children also are at risk, since their parents may not be able to take them for checkups. Since fluoridated water is not usually available in rural communities, the need for transportation for regular dental checkups and care is even greater. Transportation challenges are not confined to rural areas; however, public transportation is not readily available or completely lacking in many rural areas.

## A Call to Action

There is consensus that a successful intervention to correct these deficits in oral care must take a comprehensive approach, with immediate and rigorous attention to enhancing dental service capacity, expanding the pool of dental providers, broadening the scope of the dental skills of locally available providers, creating new interdisciplinary teams, and developing a more comprehensive oral care policy (Beetstra et al., 2002). But the first step is to change perceptions so that oral health becomes accepted as an integral component of general health, an effort which will require dramatic change across all disciplines within the health-care system.

Based on the literature review and the insight that we have gained through our collective experience in the health care field, the following recommendations related to practice, education and policy development are offered for consideration.

- Promote daily oral care. Effective daily oral care is the most crucial factor in oral health, and must receive the same priority as other health care practices. It is imperative that physicians, nurses, and other health care providers be better educated in oral health care, and that they view themselves and are viewed by others as an integral part of the team that promotes the public's oral health care. Standards and protocols for daily oral care, as well as tools to assess oral health status in remote areas, must be developed by multidisciplinary teams and implemented daily with the persons they serve.
- Develop oral health policies. Policymakers must develop more comprehensive oral health policies and adequate mechanisms for dental coverage, supported by grass roots organizations, institutional priorities, and local and national government agencies.
- Forge partnerships. Public-private partnerships must be forged to remove barriers between people and the services needed to improve oral health.
- Study oral health issues. There is continuing need for research to inform us about the deficits in oral health, particularly in at-risk and underserved segments of the population, and to examine personal, educational, clinical, and political issues relevant to oral health. There also is a pressing need for continued research into breakthrough techniques to boost

prevention and treatment, as fluoridation of water did in the 1940s.
- Coordinate efforts with accepted national dental organizations such as the American Dental Association (ADA) and the Academy of General Dentistry (AGD).

## *Removing Barriers to Access for Oral Care*

The remainder of this discussion will describe actions that have been taken in several states to overcome barriers to the oral health of their citizens. Several predominantly rural states have instituted innovative changes that are starting to improve access to dental care for their residents. For example, Alabama has improved its access to oral health care services for Medicaid-eligible children through their *Smile Alabama!* Program (Greene-McIntyre, Finch, & Searcy, 2003). Fiscal year 1999 data taken prior to this initiative showed that only 26% of the children enrolled in Alabama Medicaid received any dental services, 19 out of 67 counties in Alabama had one or no Medicaid-participating dental provider, and only 11% of dentists in Alabama were accepting new Medicaid patients. In response to surveys from the dental community, this multi-agency collaboration targeted claims processing, dental reimbursement, provider education and recruitment, and recipient education (p. 407). As a result, by fiscal year 2002 the total number of children receiving dental services had increased by 57%, the number of counties with one or no Medicaid provider had decreased to 10 and the number of participating dental providers had increased by 38%.

States have placed a major emphasis on expanding the pool of dental providers who are willing to serve indigent and uninsured populations. To encourage participation, several states have recently instituted Medicaid dental reimbursement rates that are marketplace-driven and approach the 75th to 85th percentile of the fee schedules, based on zip codes, that insurance companies will pay for their subscribers. In other words, the outdated and inadequate Medicaid fee schedules in these states have been converted to ones based on a percentage of "usual and customary" charges. Some states also have lessened the administrative burden associated with billing. As a result, significantly more dental providers participate in the Medicaid program in these states, and enrollees have gained improved access to locally available dental providers.

Addressing the need for physicians to be better educated relative to oral health, the Department of Family Medicine at the University of Kentucky Medical Center developed a curriculum to teach family medicine residents to perform oral health screening and risk assessment and to recognize and manage common oral conditions for children ages five years and under (Gonsalves et al., 2004).

In New Mexico, a group of concerned providers, academicians, legislators, public health officials, and other oral health stakeholders collaborated in seeking solutions to the dental crisis (Beetstra et al., 2002). They incorporated oral health services into a "health commons" model, in which resources from public and private entities are pooled to address complex health issues that cannot be solved by any single entity alone. The enhanced health commons sites include medical, nursing, behavioral, social, public, and oral health services, in accessible community-based sites. One of their projects involved incorporating dental hygienists into primary care clinics. Working under the supervision of the medical director of each primary care facility, the hygienist functioned as part of the primary care team. Preventive dental services are provided at the same time as routine medical care, increasing access for many at-risk persons, including young children, seniors, and people with chronic medical problems such as diabetes and heart disease. While this model was first tested in urban settings, it would seem to have utility in rural settings, as well.

## *Addressing the Shortage of Dental Providers in Rural Communities*

A number of primarily rural states also have taken steps to address the shortage of dental providers in remote communities. Virtually all states have initiated attractive loan repayment programs and scholarships to recruit dental graduates to underserved areas. Other innovative multidisciplinary programs and policy changes have also been initiated, as described below.

## No-Cost Licensing for Retired Dental Professionals

Wyoming is considering legislation to extend health care to underserved populations by allowing retired dentists and dental hygienists, as well as physicians, nurses, physician's assistants, and pharmacists to obtain volunteer licenses to treat uninsured low-income patients in not-for-profit care facilities. Volunteer licenses would be provided without cost and would be renewable annually (Krause et al., 2003). It follows that malpractice insurance would need to be offered at no cost to these dental volunteers.

## Less Restrictive Practice Model for Dental Hygienists

Given the extreme shortage of dentists, a number of states have taken steps to change the traditional legal requirement that dental hygienists must practice under the direct supervision of a dentist, seeking policy revisions that allow them to practice under primary care physicians in geographically defined shortage areas, institutions, homes, and in mobile practices. Seventeen states have adopted this less restrictive health policy model, or are using this model in pilot programs, which permits dental hygienists to perform all duties except removing irreversible tooth structure or soft tissue (Krause et al., 2003) under the supervision of primary care physicians.

## Introducing Oral Education and Services into Community Settings

Teaching young children preventive strategies that reduce oral disease prepares them to adopt long-term behaviors to maintain oral and overall health. Accordingly, there is a move to introduce actual preventive dental services broadly into publicly funded elementary schools and day care facilities in rural areas. Similar innovative models of service are being developed for long term care and rehabilitation facilities (Krause et al., 2003).

## Expanding Dental Skills of Non-Dental Health Providers

In sparsely populated states, the problem of access is greatly magnified by a shortage and an uneven geographic distribution of dentists and other oral health providers (Beetstra et al., 2002, p. 12). Addressing this problem, the University of New Mexico instituted a teaching program to expand the dental skills of other health providers in the community i.e., family physicians, emergency room residents, and dental hygienists. Graduates of the program are able to perform emergency dental procedures in rural emergency departments (p. 13). In addition, a relationship was established with several remote communities to provide local dental services, and to update the skills of local providers.

## Teledentistry

The Children's Hospital Los Angeles Teledentistry Project, operated in association with the University of Southern California Mobile Dental Clinic, seeks to increase and enhance the quality of oral health care that is provided to children living in remote rural areas of California, areas often severely underserved by dental health providers (Chang et al., 2003). Prescreening of children and the creation of an electronic medical record with health histories and digital oral radiographs allows for efficient, cost-effective care during visits by the mobile dental clinic.

## A County Approach

Tioga County, in rural upstate New York, has instituted a comprehensive county-wide program to prevent dental disease, with oral health education and preventive dental services provided by a dental health coordinator, dental hygienists, and a dental assistant. This county-wide oral health education program offers screening, oral health education, parent education, dental nutrition classes, and oral cancer education to children and adults at various sites throughout the county, including schools, preschools, community centers, work sites, and health fairs. Fluoride prescriptions or supplements are available for children from birth to age 12. The school-based program offers dental assessment, sealants, and referrals for treatment for children grades two though six, and weekly fluoride rinses for students in grades K–8. In 2003 a mobile dental van was outfitted to provide dental care for children in 12 school districts and at a community center. In 2004, over 3,000 persons received dental education, over 1,200 received an oral health assessment, and over 700 children received sealants (Tioga County Health Department, 2004).

Neighboring Broome County in upstate New York was designated a Dental Health Care Professional Shortage Area for the low income population in 2004. As the result of the critical community need, the Broome County Health Department partnered with Our Lady of Lourdes Hospital to obtain funding through the New York State Department of Health's Innovative Dental Services Grant to establish the Lourdes Center for Oral Care. The Center provides dental care to low-income children and their families and is in the process of procuring a mobile dental office to provide services at schools and various community sites. Services provided include prophylaxis, urgent care, patient education, fluoride treatments, dental treatments, X-rays, and sealants. Restorations, extractions and exams are performed by the dentists who participate in the initiative, and the other services are provided by dental hygienists. Since the Center for Oral Health opened in January of 2005, they have had about 3,000 patient visits and have enrolled 3,700 patients in the program in the first six months (Lucy Bianco, personal communication, June 23, 2005).

## *Responding to the Surgeon General's Mandate*

The Surgeon General's report (USDHHS, 2000) indicates that physicians have the opportunity to identify oral health problems in children seven times more frequently than do dentists in the first three years of life; however, studies show that education related to oral health is still lacking in most medical school curricula. Consequently, few physicians are trained to recognize, treat, or refer children to dental health providers (Mouradian et al., 2003; Mouradian et al., 2000). The report also acknowledges that there are profound and consequential disparities in the oral health of our nation's citizens (USDHHS, 2000, p. vii). Those who suffer the worst oral health are found among the poor of all ages, with poor children and elders at greatest risk. Members of minority groups are also at disproportionate risk for oral health problems. Poor families often do not have the money to pay for dental care out of pocket and may not have dental insurance. Fewer people have dental insurance than have medical insurance, and insurance coverage is often lost when older individuals retire (p. vii). Public dental insurance programs such as Medicaid are often inadequate. Many poor and minority citizens lack transportation to a clinic or can not get time off from work to access services. For some, "disparities are exacerbated by the lack of programs such as fluoridated water supplies" (p. vii). Another major barrier to seeking and obtaining professional oral health care is the lack of public understanding and awareness of the importance or oral health (USDHHS, 2000).

"The report proposes solutions that entail partnerships — government agencies and officials, private industry, foundations, consumer groups, health professionals, educators, and researchers to co-ordinate and facilitate actions based on a *National Oral Health Plan*" (USDHHS, 2000, iii). The report also emphasized the importance of facilitating collaborations to enhance education, service, and research in order to eliminate barriers to oral care.

In recent years, research findings have demonstrated the impact of oral health on quality of life and general health (New York State Department of Health, 2005). The experience of pain, endurance of dental abscesses, problems with eating, and embarrassment about missing, discolored, or damaged teeth adversely affects people's daily lives, self-esteem and well-being. It has also been pointed out that failure to attend to oral health in children can have a negative impact on the child's self-image and ability to learn and seek employment as an adult (Gift, Reisine, & Larach, 1992).

## Research Implications

As a nation, we do not have adequate information about oral health practices and care for diverse segments of the population, including underserved rural populations. Health services research is needed to provide critical information about the cost, cost-effectiveness, and outcomes of treatment (USDHHS, 2000, p. 284).

## *A Framework for Action*

To address the problem of poor oral health in this country, we suggest a three-pronged approach that targets the public, policymakers and healthcare providers:

1. We must initiate an educational awareness program to change the public's perception that oral disorders are less important than other illnesses.
2. We must inform policymakers about the importance of oral health, and engage them in an effort to ensure inclusion of oral health services in all health promotion and disease prevention programs, care delivery systems, and reimbursement schedules (USDHHS, 2000, p. 11). Two of the most pressing tasks are to develop oral health policies related to Medicaid reimbursement and to increase the role of the dental hygienist to be able to perform all legal clinical procedures permitted within respective state regulations, enabling them to significantly increase preventive oral health and screening at the community level.
3. We must change the perception of non-dental health providers that oral care is someone else's responsibility. "Too little time is devoted to oral health and disease topics in the education of nondental health professionals" (USDHHS, 2000, p. 11). All healthcare providers should contribute to improving oral health. This can best be accomplished by including oral health content as a part of the curricula of all health professions, so that primary care providers across disciplines will know how to evaluate oral health, advise patients in matters of oral health promotion, and refer patients to oral health practitioners for more complex oral problems.

## Summary

Poor oral health is an increasingly common problem in our country, particularly among poor and minority citizens. Poor oral health has a significant impact on general health status and overall well-being (USDHHS, 2000, p. 4). Barriers to adequate care include lack of dental insurance, reimbursement issues and inaccessibility to oral health services, especially for persons who live in remote areas and may not have transportation to travel for care. Oral health also seems to be given low priority when compared to non-dental health issues, both among the general public and healthcare providers (Glover, Moore, Samuels, & Probst, 2004).

While there are many barriers to achieving optimal oral health, there seems to be growing consensus that the key to reversing this trend rests in the formation of multidisciplinary community-based networks that include not only dentists and dental hygienists, but also nurses, physicians, nutritionists, social workers, community organizations, private businesses, policymakers, families and individuals. We tend to think of our country as the most technologically advanced and civilized in the world, yet we seem to be decades late in confronting this basic health care need for our citizens. The time to correct this inequitable situation is *now*.

## REFERENCES

Allender, J. A., & Spradley, B. W. (2001). *Community health nursing: Concepts and practice* (5th ed.). Philadelphia, PA: Lippincott, Williams & Wilkins.

Beetstra, S., Derksen, D., Ro, M., Powell, W., Fry, D. E., & Kaufman, A. (2002). A "health commons" approach to oral health for low-income populations in a rural state. *Am J Public Health*, 92(1), 12–13.

The Centers for Disease Control and Prevention [CDC]. (2001). Recommendations for using fluoride to prevent and control dental caries in the United States. *Morbidity and Mortality Weekly Report*, 50(RR 14), v, 42 p.

Chang, S. W., Plotkin, D. R., Mulligan, R., Polido, J. C., Mah, J. K., & Meara, J. G. (2003). Teledentistry in rural california: A USC Initiative. *J Calif Dent Assoc*, 31(8), 601–608.

Ebersole, P., Hess, P., & Luggen, A. S. (2003). *Toward healthy aging: Human needs and nursing response* (6th, Revised ed.). Philadelphia: Mosby; Elsevier — Health Sciences Division.

Fitzpatrick, J. (2000). Oral health care needs of dependent older people: Responsibilities of nurses and care staff. *J Adv Nurs*, 32(6), 1325–1332.

Gift, H. C., Reisine, S. T., & Larach, D. C. (1992). The social impact of dental problems and visits. *Am J Public Health*, 82(12), 1663–1668.

Glover, S., Moore, C. G., Samuels, M. E., & Probst, J. C. (2004). Disparities in access to care among rural working-age adults. *J Rural Health*, 20(3), 193–205.

Gonsalves, W. C., Skelton, J., Smith, T., Hardison, D., & Ferretti, G. (2004). Physicians' oral health education in Kentucky. *Fam Med*, 36(8), 544–546.

Greene-McIntyre, M., Finch, M. H., & Searcy, J. (2003). Smile Alabama! initiative: Interim results from a program to increase children's access to dental care. *J Rural Health*, 19 Suppl, 407–415.

Heaton, L. J., Smith, T. A., & Raybould, T. P. (2004). Factors influencing use of dental services in rural and urban communities: Considerations for practitioners in underserved areas. *J Dent Educ*, 68(10), 1081–1089.

Hobbins, M. (1999). Oral health of the cognitively impaired person: An interdisciplinary responsibility. In S. H. Gueldner & L. W. Poon (Eds.), *Gerontological nursing issues for the 21st century: A multidisciplinary dialogue commemorating the international year of older persons* (pp. 99–103.). Washington, DC: Center Nursing.

Janes, G., Blackman, D., Bolen, J., Kamimoto, L., Rhodes, L., Caplan, L., et al. (1999). Surveillance for use of preventive health-care services by older adults. In *CDC Surveillance Summaries December 17, 1999 MMRW* (Vol. 48, pp. 51–88). Atlanta: USDHHS, Epidemiology Program Office, CDC.

Jensen, G. L., Friedmann, J. M., Coleman, C. D., & Smiciklas-Wright, H. (2001). Screening for hospitalization and nutritional risks among community-dwelling older persons. *Am J Clin Nutr*, 74(2), 201–205.

Krause, D., Mosca, N., & Livingston, M. (2003). Maximizing the dental workforce: Implications for a rural state. *J Dent Hyg*, 77(4), 253–261.

Mouradian, W. E., Schaad, D., Kim, S., Leggott, P., Domoto, P., Maier, R., et al. (2003). Addressing disparities in children's oral health: A dental-medical partnership to train family practice residents. *J Dent Educ*, 67(8), 886–895.

Mouradian, W. E., Wehr, E., & Crall, J. J. (2000). Disparities in children's oral health and access to dental care. *JAMA*, 284(20), 2625–2631.

National Center for Chronic Disease Prevention and Health Promotion [NCCDPHP]. (2001). *Oral Health for Older Americans*: CDC.

National Center for Chronic Disease Prevention and Health Promotion [NCCDPHP]. (2002). *HHS agencies team with Academy of General Dentistry to promote Healthy People 2010 oral health objectives*. Retrieved August 7, 2005, from http://www.cdc.gov/oralhealth/pressreleases/healthy_people.htm

National Center for Chronic Disease Prevention and Health Promotion [NCCDPHP]. (2006a). *Oral Health for Adults*: CDC.

National Center for Chronic Disease Prevention and Health Promotion [NCCDPHP]. (2006b). *Oral Health for Older Americans*: CDC.

New York State Department of Health. (1992). *NYCRR Title 10 Section 415.17 Dental Services*: Author.

New York State Department of Health. (2005). *Oral Health Plan for New York State*. Albany: Author.

NIDCR. (2006). *Periodontal (gum) disease: Causes, symptoms, and treatments*. Retrieved August 7, 2005 & Jan 20, 2006, 2006, from http://www.nidcr.nih.gov

Petersen, P. E., & Yamamoto, T. (2005). Improving the oral health of older people: The approach of the WHO Global Oral Health Programme. *Community Dentistry and Oral Epidemiology*, 33(2), 81–92.

Roberts, J. (2000). Developing an oral assessment and intervention tool for older people: 3. *Br J Nurs*, 9(19), 2073–2078.

Tioga County Health Department. (2004). Annual Report: 2004.

United States Department of Health and Human Services [USDHHS]. (2000). *Oral health in America a report of the surgeon general*, from http://purl.access.gpo.gov/GPO/LPS13826

United States Department of Health and Human Services [USDHHS]. (2005). *Financing dental education: Public policy interests, issues and strategic considerations,*

2006, from http://bhpr.hrsa.gov/healthworkforce/reports/dental/default.htm, ftp://ftp.hrsa.gov/bhpr/nationalcenter/dental.pdf

Vargas, C. M., Kramarow, E. A., & Yellowitz, J. A. (2001). The oral health of older Americans. *Aging Trends, 3,* 1–8.

Vargus, C. M., Yellowitz, J., & Hayes, K. (2003). Oral health status of older rural adults in the United States. *J Am Dent Assoc, 134*(4), 479–486.

Wardh, I., Hallberg, L. R., Berggren, U., Andersson, L., & Sorensen, S. (2000). Oral health care — a low priority in nursing: In-depth interviews with nursing staff. *Scand J Caring Sci, 14*(2), 137–142.

*Chapter 4*

# Health Maintenance Flow Sheet for Agricultural Workers

### LINDSAY LAKE MORGAN

## Introduction

In the United States, there are well-established recommendations for periodic health screening developed for age groups, but none for occupational groups. Government agencies, unions, and/or employers oversee the health and safety of many workers. This is not true, however, for many agricultural workers in the U.S. who are often self-employed, work alone, and/or are not subject to government involvement. Further, limited access to health care in rural areas creates an environment in which primary care providers have less opportunity to conduct office visits that focus on primary prevention of health problems. Given the need for health and safety for agricultural workers and few opportunities for assessment and teaching, this paper proposes a Health Maintenance Flow Sheet for primary health care providers whose clientele are agricultural workers. The recommendations in the flow sheet were developed from health risks described in the literature.

## Prevention, Screening, and Health Counseling/Education

In our current atmosphere of increasing preventive services, controlling health care costs, and increasing patient responsibility for their own health, the United States Preventive Services Task Force urges health care providers to provide:

- Screening tests — for early detection of pre-clinical conditions or risk factors
- Education/Counseling interventions — to educate about consequences of personal health behaviors
- Immunizations — to prevent infectious diseases
- Chemoprophylaxis — by asymptomatic people to prevent future disease

Health care providers in farming-dependent areas are confronted with distinct challenges in delivering health promotion and disease prevention to agricultural workers. This article will highlight the health care needs that are significant to agricultural workers and guide the provider in delivering preventive services. The Health Maintenance Flow Sheet is intended to inform office staff and providers of the screening and health care needs of the agricultural worker. It can serve as a communication tool among health professionals. Specific problems within a region may emerge with the consistent use of the tool as part of established surveillance mechanisms. The flow sheet also has the potential to provide epidemiological data to guide health professionals in selecting continuing education programs and preparing health education for the community. The challenges in providing health promotion and disease prevention for agricultural workers are related to both the individuals receiving care and the health care providers. Awareness of these challenges will encourage creative locally appropriate solutions.

## *Agricultural Workers*

Farm workers experience distinct risks for illness and injury and barriers to accessing care. Health promotion and disease prevention are only beginning to achieve general acceptance among agricultural workers and are even further compromised by the nature of the agricultural lifestyle.

### *Barriers to Preventive Care for Agricultural Workers*

Agricultural Workers

- Seek health care for acute problems rather than for health maintenance.

## Health Maintenance Flow Sheet for Agricultural Workers

- May experience limitations to health care such as finances, insurance, geography, and work burden.
- May lack work site health programs due to small size of business and self-employment.

### Acute Care versus Health Maintenance

Farmers define health as "the ability to work" (Long & Weinert, 1989). Dairy farmers in particular are not able to be absent at milking time unless other, often expensive, arrangements are made. Because farmers may be indispensable to their work, they push themselves to work when they are ill or injured. They will seek health care only when they are unable to ignore the health problem. Under these circumstances, farmers often seek health care in almost an emergency state. Sometimes they need a higher level of care because of waiting until the health problem compelled action. As a result, health maintenance, disease/injury prevention, and health education are low priorities at health care visits.

### Limitations

Since they are self-employed, farmers may forego buying health insurance for themselves and their families due to the expense. Further, there is no law that requires farmers as employers to insure their workers. Lack of insurance also may inhibit farm workers from seeking health care. As noted above, visits for health care may be limited to emergencies only. Finances are often constrained and a machine needing a part will take precedence over health problems that do not interfere with work. Some types of farming do not allow for absences while tending to one's personal health. Rural places are often designated as medically underserved areas for primary care and the ability to access specialty care may be extremely limited for the farm worker and their families. Geography, distance, and poor roads are other potential barriers to seeking health care.

## Lack of Work Site Health Care

The Occupational Safety and Health Administration [OSHA] has jurisdiction over employers of ten or more workers, but 97% percent of U.S. farms are below this criterion (Steven Stockdale, personal communication, September 1999). Therefore, there are no occupational safety and health standards for farmers to meet; nor are there recommendations to assist them in protecting themselves. OSHA has proposed a new safety and health program rule requiring hazard identification and assessment, hazard prevention and control, information and training, and evaluation for all employers EXCEPT those engaged in construction and agriculture (OSHA, 2003).

On-site health care is mandatory in American industry only if there are no adequate health care services "nearby." By this standard, it seems that farms would be the most appropriate place for on-site health care. However, 97% of farms, as noted above, are not included in this standard. Health care on farms has limited feasibility. An alternative is the provision of preventative education by primary care providers.

## Rural Health Care Providers

Rural health care providers experience difficulties providing health promotion and disease prevention to agricultural workers because of limitations in preparation and delivery.

### Difficulties of Rural Health Care Provision

Preparation

- May not be educated in rural health.
- Do not have specialty education in the health concerns of agricultural workers.
- Have difficulty obtaining any continuing education due to issues of distance and isolation.
- Do not find continuing education related to the topic of rural health.

Delivery

- Are often practicing in underserved areas and are overburdened.
- May have office personnel who need guidance in patient teaching.
- May share a practice with multiple providers, requiring effective communication.

## *Preparation*

Rural health is a new area of study and the literature is just beginning to grow. Few universities are offering courses in rural health. Most primary providers have not had the opportunity to study specific agricultural health problems such as zoonotic diseases or the respiratory diseases related to agricultural exposures. In addition to the developing literature base, many websites on the Internet provide helpful information and some continuing education offerings are addressing this special population. However, the provider must be highly motivated to seek out these sparse and less convenient resources.

## *Delivery*

Rural health care providers are often practicing in underserved areas and are overburdened. The burden is a result of few providers, limited specialties, limited hospital support, a large and/or challenging geographic area, and diverse populations representing varied needs. Such a burden requires efficiency during visits and guidance with rural health problems. Office staff as well may be carrying out several different roles within the practice. One individual, with limited health care education may serve as receptionist, transcriptionist, billing clerk, nurse, technician, and patient educator among other roles. Finally, some practices use itinerant providers or rotation among several clinics. This is a useful way of supplying non-urgent specialty visits to a large area. The client record is the form of communication among various providers and must be effective and efficient.

## The Agricultural Worker Health Maintenance Flow Sheet

The Agricultural Worker Health Maintenance Flow Sheet is adjunct to the routine adult health screening/maintenance schedules recommended in existing protocols such as those from the United States Preventive Services Task Force or the Canadian Task Force on Preventive Health Care. For example, the U.S. Preventive Services Task Force [USPSTF] (USPSTF, 1995) provides age-specific charts suggesting screening, counseling, immunizations, and chemoprophylaxis for the general population and interventions for high-risk populations. After assuring the basic measures have been met for each client, the content on the Agricultural Worker Flow Sheet (Appendix A) can be addressed.

### *Screening Tests*

The WHO criteria for screening for disease are as follows:
1. The condition sought should be an important health problem for the individual and community.
2. There should be an accepted treatment or useful intervention for patients with the disease.
3. The natural history of the disease should be adequately understood.
4. There should be a latent or early symptomatic stage.
5. There should be a suitable and acceptable screening test or examination.
6. Facilities for diagnosis and treatment should be available.
7. There should be an agreed policy on whom to treat as patients.
8. Treatment started at an early stage should be of more benefit than treatment started later.
9. The cost should be economically balanced in relation to possible expenditure on medical care as a whole.
10. Case finding should be a continuing process and not a once and for all project. (Wilson & Jungner, 1968, pp. 26–27)

Agricultural workers are at increased risk for the certain health problems. For some health problems, there are cost-effective screenings that can easily be conducted during an office visit. Other problems should be kept in mind when evaluating an agricultural worker because there are no screens or testing available does not meet criteria for screening. In some cases it has not yet been determined whether the criteria are met. This is the case because of the first criterion. If one considers agricultural workers a community — then certain health conditions may be considered important enough for this population to warrant screening, but not important enough to screen the general population. Screening "at-risk" populations is an accepted practice. Screenings to consider for the agricultural worker are: alcohol use, audiometry, selected cancers, depression, focused neurological exam, pulmonary function testing, skin exam, and domestic violence.

## *Health Counseling and Education*

Health counseling and education are more successful when they are targeted to the population to be served. A provider should learn the risks that are common to the types of farming in the area and evaluate the barriers to healthy behaviors. Because of the brief and focused nature of health care visits as discussed above, providers may wish to become a health information resource for the community by informing through other channels. These might include 4-H, Patrons of Husbandry (Grange), Rotary Club, Radio/TV spots, schools, or a web site. Strategies that succeed with adult learners include providing handouts, describing how the safety behaviors will help them perform better, and associating changes directly with results that can be expected in the near future. Important counseling/education topics for agricultural workers suggested by the literature are listed on the flow sheet and include safety issues, prevention of injury and exposures, and general healthy behaviors.

## *Immunizations and Chemoprophylaxis*

Immunization recommendations are not different for agricultural workers but may require more vigilance because of the nature of their work. Chemoprophylaxis, specifically the use of sunscreen is an obvious necessity for agricultural workers who are outdoors for their livelihoods. However, adherence to this recommendation is difficult for many reasons (Marlenga, 1995; Robinson et al., 2004). Robinson and colleagues did find that providers' counseling can positively affect preventive behaviors.

## Summary

In response to the barriers to preventive care for agricultural workers, a Health Maintenance Flow Sheet is proposed. The flow sheet, used over time, will make a routine of health maintenance through the review of a checklist at every visit. Since visits may be infrequent, the use of the flow sheet is efficient and thorough. It would prevent repetition while assuring attention to common agricultural worker risks. The education suggested on the flow sheet is similar to that provided by on-site programs in other industries.

Use of the Agricultural Worker Health Maintenance Flow Sheet can help resolve both the preparation and delivery problems for rural health care providers. Until rural health education resources are more prevalent and accessible, the flow sheet gives a provider a starting place to evaluate the risks and needs in the geographic region served. As the provider identifies new areas of concern for the service population, they can be added to the flow sheet. In this way, the flow sheet can support continuing education by identifying needs. Research and case finding can be established from the flow sheet record.

During limited visits with agricultural workers, the Health Maintenance Flow Sheet can increase efficiency for providing maintenance and risk reduction. It serves as a record of health education issues, when it was accomplished, and who completed it. If all staff consults the Agricultural Worker Health Maintenance Flow Sheet, continuity of care can be assured.

Agricultural workers have responsibility for their own health, but are lacking opportunities for guidance in safe, healthy behaviors. Barriers to preventive care for farm workers include seeking health care for acute problems rather than for health maintenance, limitations such as finances, insurance, geography, and work burden, and the lack of work-site health programs. Rural health care providers also have trouble providing such care to farm workers related to preparation and health care delivery. The Agricultural Worker Health Maintenance Flow Sheet was developed in response to the barriers and limitations that obscure superior health care. The flow sheet implements the United States Preventive Services Task Force Guidelines by addressing screening, counseling/education, immunizations, and chemoprophylaxis. Providers can respond to the learning and health needs of farm workers in an organized, comprehensive manner by using the flow sheet at every visit. Ultimately, a large sample of flow sheets can be analyzed to uncover the most pressing health concerns among agricultural workers in a service region.

## REFERENCES

Long, K. A. & Weinert, C. (1989). Rural nursing: Developing the theory base. *Scholarly Inquiry for Nursing Practice*, 3, 113–127.

Marlenga, B. (1995). The health beliefs and skin cancer prevention practices of Wisconsin dairy farmers. *Oncology Nursing Forum*, 22(4), 681–686.

OSHA. (2003). Draft proposed safety and health program rule. http://www.osha.gov/SLTC/safetyhealth/nshp.html Accessed 4/22/2003.

Robinson, J. D., Silk, K. J., Parrott, R. L., Steiner, C., Morris, S. M., Honeycutt, C. (2004). Healthcare providers' sun-protection promotion and at-risk clients' skin-cancer-prevention outcomes. *Preventive Medicine*, 38(3), 251–257.

USPSTF. (1995). *Guide to Clinical Preventive Services*, (2nd ed.). Department of Health and Human Services, Office of Public Health and Science, Office of Disease Prevention and Health Promotion, U.S. Preventive Services Task Force.

Wilson, J. M. G. & Jungner, G. (1968). *Principles and Practice of Screening for Disease*. Geneva: World Health Organization.

## Occupational Health Flow Sheet – Agricultural Worker

Name _____  Date of Birth _____

| Date→ | | | | | | | | | | |
|---|---|---|---|---|---|---|---|---|---|---|
| **Screening Tests** O = Ordered  N = Result Normal  A = Result Abnormal  R = Refused  E = Done Elsewhere | | | | | | | | | | |
| Alcohol use (CAGE) | | | | | | | | | | |
| Audiometry | | | | | | | | | | |
| Cancer | | | | | | | | | | |
| Depression Scale | | | | | | | | | | |
| Neurological Exam | | | | | | | | | | |
| Pulmonary Function Testing | | | | | | | | | | |
| Skin Examination | | | | | | | | | | |
| Domestic Violence | | | | | | | | | | |
| | | | | | | | | | | |
| **Education** D = Discussed  E = Evaluated  P = Pamphlet  R = Reinforced  NR = Needs Reinforcement  N/A = Not Applicable  Level of Understanding  1 = no understanding  2 = moderate understanding  3 = understands | | | | | | | | | | |
| Animal Infectious Disease | | | | | | | | | | |
| Animal Injury | | | | | | | | | | |
| Carcinogens | | | | | | | | | | |
| Children – safety | | | | | | | | | | |
| Equipment – safety | | | | | | | | | | |
| Finances | | | | | | | | | | |
| Firearm safety | | | | | | | | | | |
| Stress | | | | | | | | | | |
| Food storage on the job | | | | | | | | | | |
| Handling Laundry | | | | | | | | | | |
| Hearing protection | | | | | | | | | | |
| Lung protection | | | | | | | | | | |
| Musculoskeletal safety/Body mechanics | | | | | | | | | | |
| Nutrition | | | | | | | | | | |
| Exercise | | | | | | | | | | |
| Emergency measures | | | | | | | | | | |
| Skin protection | | | | | | | | | | |
| Thermo regulation | | | | | | | | | | |
| Wounds | | | | | | | | | | |
| | | | | | | | | | | |
| **Immunizations** | | | | | | | | | | |
| Tetanus Booster | | | | | | | | | | |
| | | | | | | | | | | |
| **Chemoprophylaxis** | | | | | | | | | | |
| Sunscreen | | | | | | | | | | |
| | | | | | | | | | | |

© Lindsay Lake Morgan 2007

*Chapter 5*

# Sustaining Geriatric Rural Populations

JOHN A. KROUT AND MARILYN KINNER

## Introduction

In 2000, 8.3 million or 24% of the 65 years and older population lived in non-metropolitan areas (Golant, 2003). Data on non-metropolitan counties are very often used to describe and analyze "rural" life and this practice is not without problems, to be addressed later in this paper. It is not surprising that more rural states have larger percentages of their older population living in rural places particularly in the Midwest, South, and a few New England states. Two-thirds of Vermont's older population lives in rural places, while the figure for New Jersey is only 10%. More populous states tend to have the largest number of rural elders: (a) Texas, (b) Pennsylvania, and (c) North Carolina. In general, the more rural a community, the greater the percent of population that is 65 years of age and over. Nationally this percent was 14.7% for non-metropolitan counties and 11.9% for metropolitan counties (U.S. Census Bureau, 2001). So, almost all states face questions about how rurality impacts the lives of older people and responses to their health and social needs. In New York State, counties of less than 200,000 in total population are defined as rural (Eberts and Merschrod, 2003). These counties had 450,000 persons ages 65 and over, about 15% of the population.

It is important to note that with some exceptions, many rural areas have recently experienced very small gains or even a loss in population and resources. Most rural counties had about 14% of their population age 65 and over in 2000, higher than the statewide average of close to 13% (Eberts and Merschrod, 2003). In addition, declines in access to health and economic services, corporate centralization in health care, changes in health care delivery and policy, such as managed care, have all constricted the availability of acute care in rural areas. Low population densities and inadequate funding of community-based care services combine to reduce the number and types of care options available to older adults and their families. Twentieth-century transportation changes, air and surface, increasingly have left rural America behind. For economically and socially advantaged rural elders, these things are not so problematic. For disadvantaged rural elders, they can significantly impact quality of life.

## What is Rural?

Like the older population in general, rural elders are very diverse in their characteristics and needs and live in a variety of communities, each with its unique set of resources and problems. Rural elders live in communities that can be typified in many ways such as: (a) farming; (b) ranching; (c) mining; (d) manufacturing; (e) retirement in-migration; (f) urban "bedroom"; (g) mixed economy; (h) stagnant or depopulating; and (i) recreation (Golant, 2003). We should note that while very few older rural adults live on farms today, many more have had connections to agriculture at some point in their lives. Perhaps the best way to understand how living in rural areas affects aging is to identify salient aspects of rurality (Krout, 1998). These include:

1. ecological — population size and density, distance from service centers, smaller "markets";
2. economic — occupations, income, poverty, cost of living;
3. culture and lifestyle — values, health risks; and
4. community organization — resource mobilization, social organizations, political clout.

Almost all research on rural aging uses ecological indicators to define a place or person as being rural. The simplest and most widespread definition of rural is any county not in a metropolitan county. Thus, "non-metropolitan" and "rural" are often used interchangeably even though the Census Bureau definition of rural is any place of less than 2,500 in population. The metropolitan/non-metropolitan designation has some advantages, but it is a very gross measure that lumps all kinds of places together and therefore obscures much of the variation found within the two categories. Indeed, rural observers are often fond of saying, "If you have seen one rural community, you have seen one rural community." One option is to use continuums that combine factors such as population size and/or density and relative location of counties in a population size hierarchy. Noted below is one such continuum (Golant, 2003).

1. Large — central and fringe counties of large metropolitan areas of 1 million or more.
2. Small — counties in small metropolitan areas of fewer than 1 million population.
3. Adjacent to a large metropolitan area with a city of 10,000 or more.
4. Adjacent to a large metropolitan area with a city of at least 10,000.
5. Adjacent to a small metropolitan area with a city of 10,000 or more.
6. Adjacent to a small metropolitan area without a city of 10,000 or more.
7. Not adjacent to a metropolitan area and with a city of 10,000 or more.
8. Not adjacent to a metropolitan area and with a city of 2,500 to 9,999 population.
9. Not adjacent to a metropolitan area and with no city or a city with a population less than 2,500.

The importance of population size, density, and relative location, for understanding aging is in how they impact or are related to the factors that are known to effect health and well-being, needs, and the ability of communities to provide for those needs. For example, older people living in smaller, more remote areas may have fewer individual economic resources because their earnings have been lower throughout their lives and they have fewer local opportunities to work in old age. Small towns experiencing economic decline or stagnation often see an out-migration of young adults reducing the availability of proximate family caregivers such as adult children. Smaller populations are also less able to support an adequate amount and variety of health care services or housing options.

## Characteristics of Rural Elders

The diversity of rural communities supports equally diverse rural older populations. So, no one profile of this population is accurate or can be relied upon for program planning or practice. Having said this, national data do suggest some important observations about who rural elders are. In general, rural areas compared to non-rural, have higher percents in the 65–74 and 75–84 age groups. In New York state between 1990 and 2000, rural counties had smaller increases in the under 18 and 18–44 age groups but larger increases in the 45–64 and 65+ age groups than was true state wide. Rural sex ratios are more balanced, especially in farm areas, meaning there are more older men relative to older women and rural elders are more likely to be married. Nationally, the great majority of rural elders are white, and over 90% of black rural elders live in the South. But these data should not divert us from the fact that social and racial diversity is an important aspect of rural aging, nationally and locally. Rural elders, on average, have fewer years of formal education and have significantly lower incomes (Krout, 1998).

## Myths and Realities of Rural Aging

To understand the needs of the rural elderly, we first must identify and refute the myths of rural aging (Krout, 1994a). The myths are that rural elders: (a) live on farms and are a homogenous group; (b) are in better physical and mental health due to hard work, good food, healthy rural lifestyles, and "living in the country"; (c) are more active; (d) are better able to "make ends meet" and better able to "take care of themselves"; (e) live in adequate housing — there are no "homeless"; (f) are surrounded by large and supportive kin networks that are always willing and able to help; (g) have less need for health and social services; and, (h) can get everything they need in the "country store."

The reality is far different. In fact, rural elders can be seen as facing a double jeopardy because they face the challenge of being both old and living in a rural place (Krout, 1986). Rural elders: (a) do not live on farms, with some local exceptions; (b) are very diverse; (c) have fewer recreation and leisure opportunities available to them; (d) have incomes that are 20% lower than their urban counterparts; (e) have lower Social Security payments, smaller savings, less widespread pension coverage, fewer opportunities for part-time work, and infrequent enrollment in Supplemental Security Income (SSI); (f) are more likely to own their own home, but these homes are more likely to be older and have significant substandard features; (g) have no more frequent, probably less, contact with adult children because they live further apart which can lead to problems for "long distance" care giving; (h) have diets that are too high in fat and lacking in important nutrients and limited food choices; (i) are found to be no more or less "satisfied" with their circumstances than urban elders; (j) are less healthy than metropolitan residents and are more likely to see their health as poor; (k) have to travel further for every day goods and services; and (l) have higher rates of a number of chronic diseases among those not living on farms and more acute conditions for farm dwellers.

## *Service Deficits*

These realities are compounded by deficiencies in services (Krout, 1994a, 1998). Rural areas generally: (a) are more likely to be dependent on Medicaid as a source of payment for health care; (b) have a much lower ratio of health care professional and health services per population than found in urban places, including Medical Doctors (MD), Registered Nurses (RN), Occupational Therapists (OT), etc.; (c) have a lack of transportation for daily necessities and medical care, especially specialty care and a greater dependence on private vehicles; (d) have access to a smaller number and more narrow range of community-based services, especially services for the severely impaired; (e) have gaps in the "continuum of care"; (f) have few program models developed from evidence-based practice; and (g) have few alternatives for those who cannot live independently, but do not require institutionalization, the no care zone.

Another way to look at rural services is to list the underlying challenges facing those who would develop and provide services to rural older adults. These include service:

1. Availability: (a) insufficient number and diversity of formal services and providers; (b) shortages of qualified human and social service professionals; (c) lack of basic and high tech

equipment; (d) lack of acceptable services; and (e) general lack of human services infrastructure.
2. Accessibility: (a) access problems due to shortages of adequate, appropriate, and affordable transportation systems; (b) low population density, geographic isolation; (c) cultural and social isolation, especially of the vulnerable; (d) access problems due to terrain and weather; (e) political isolation and lack of policy input; and (f) lack of regional coordination;
3. Affordability: (a) lack of economic resources to support services, economic development, pay for match; (b) lack of economies of scale; (c) poverty and lack of income to access services, cost share; and (d) rural economics in the multi-national economy.
4. Awareness: (a) low levels of service awareness; (b) inadequate information dissemination and service referral; and (c) low levels of literacy and educational opportunities.
5. Adequacy: (a) lack of skilled professionals; (b) lack of rural standards; (c) lack of service evaluation; and (d) lack of training programs and technical assistance.
6. Acceptability: (a) traditional "rural" values, reluctance to admit need or seek help; and (b) rural reliance on self-remedies.
7. Assessment: (a) lack of information on rural programs and programming successes and failures; (b) lack of educational opportunities, training programs; and (c) lack of research, the no data zone.

These deficiencies and challenges are multi-faceted, interrelated, and result from a number of underlying issues. First are issues of priorities and funding. A lack of national interest in rural elders reflects decreased rural political clout. This results in a low priority for rural aging issues and inadequate funding for national rural health, housing, and transportation programs. Second is the lack of rural focused or sensitive education in gerontology, health, or human service training programs. Third, there is a lack of research on rural aging issues necessary to inform policy and practice and too little funding for the evaluation of the cost and effectiveness of programs serving rural elders. Finally, there is a lack of integration of existing resources at the national and state levels that can help meet rural aging needs.

## What Works?

It is useful to keep the unique characteristics of rural client populations, rural communities, and rural service systems in mind when planning any programs for rural older adults (Coward, DeWeaver, Schmidtt, & Jackson, 1983). Distinctive features of rural client populations include: (a) demographics; (b) attitudes, beliefs, and values; (c) educational attainment; (d) economic patterns; and (e) health and mental health issues. Distinctive features of rural client populations include: (a) topography and terrain; (b) population distribution; (c) cultural enclaves; (d) community organization and services; and (e) housing. Distinctive features of the provision of rural services include: (a) educational preparation and training of providers; (b) knowledge and skills of providers; (c) attributes and values of providers; and (d) task environment. We have previously noted some of these and in a number of cases, the distinctive "ruralness" of the features create real challenges for service providers and planners.

However, there are successful, very successful, programs for rural elders. While the content of these programs varies by service need, populations served, and geographic area, paying attention to the distinctive features noted above is important. Successful programs take advantage of and support community, social, cultural, and organizational systems, especially indigenous helping networks such as church, family, and neighboring. It is essential to not look at rural communities as only presenting obstacles, but to see them as also providing resources and solutions. Programs can and should be changed to fit the community, because doing otherwise is unlikely to work. Flexibility, coordination of resources, innovation, and a good dose of "common sense" are also generally required (Krout, 1994a, 2003).

Noted below are examples of successful programs identified by respondents in a national survey of area agencies on aging (Krout, 1994b):

1. Caregiver education that involves public health nurses and church parishioners.
2. Transportation using paid "volunteer" neighbors and family rather than the fixed route van approach.
3. Partnerships between schools, hospitals, and nutrition programs to lower congregate and in-home meal costs.
4. Multi-county housing coalitions that tap into federal dollars for home repair and modification.

5. Partnerships between nursing homes, senior centers, and hospitals to build congregate housing.

## *Training Rural Care Providers*

One clearly identified need in rural areas is for training in geriatric issues, especially for what are often referred to as "front line workers" such as home health and personal care aides. Over the past several years the Ithaca College Gerontology Institute has developed a program to help address this need in Central New York called "Training Rural Health Professionals: Building Capacity Through a Community Team Approach." Program support has come from the Finger Lakes Geriatric Education Center (FLGEC) and a more recent grant from the Central New York Area Health Education Center (CNYAHEC) has allowed expansion to three counties outside the Finger Lakes catchment area.

This project taps existing networks, offices for the aging, rural health networks, public health departments, departments of social services; and identifies others who have a vested interest in geriatric training such as skilled nursing facilities, home care agencies, and adult homes. It also incorporates knowledge and credibility of local professionals into the process and facilitates a geriatric training approach which strengthens the community pool of professional and paraprofessional workers. In addition the team model builds capacity for ongoing training initiated by local providers.

Initially the teams were regional encompassing two or three counties. Due to lack of time and travel constraints which prevented regional team members from participating, this approach was revised in favor of county level teams. Prospective Community Team Members in each county are identified through state agencies such as the New York State (NYS) Office for the Aging, NYS Association for Rural Health, NYS Department of Health, etc. and also through established networks. A letter outlining the FLGEC mission and the process for planning and developing a geriatric training event is sent to prospective community team members, followed by a telephone call. Teams are comprised of representatives from: (a) skilled nursing facilities; (b) home care agencies; (c) departments of public health; (d) offices for the aging; (e) rural health networks; (f) adult homes; (g) Veterans Administration (VA) medical centers; and (h) departments of social services. Team members are invited to a meeting hosted by a local agency. At this meeting local geriatric training needs are identified and prioritized. Target groups of health care and aging services professionals and paraprofessionals are identified for the chosen training topic. The format, best location, time and day for the training event are established. Barriers to developing and holding a training are also discussed.

In 2003, using this model, 14 workshops were held in 11 counties at which 719 professionals and paraprofessionals were trained. The topics addressed included:

1. Understanding and handling difficult dementia related behaviors.
2. Mental health in Long Term Care.
3. Sensitivity to age related losses.
4. Humor.
5. Stress management for professional caregivers.
6. Communication skills/conflict resolution.
7. Geriatric depression.
8. Principles of geriatric drug therapy.

## *Usefulness Survey*

Two months after the training, attendees are mailed a Usefulness Survey to ascertain whether what they learned has provided them with knowledge and skills they use in their day-to-day work with older adults. A return stamped addressed envelope is included with the survey which has resulted in an average response rate of 45%. Survey results have been very positive. These include: (a) 97.5% indicate the workshop gave them general knowledge/information that is used with clients or residents; (b) 94.2% indicate the workshop provided them with knowledge that makes them feel more confident in their work with clients or residents; (c) 96.7% indicate that it was beneficial to learn with staff from other facilities/organizations who do similar work; and (d) 94.1% shared the information with others such as co-workers, family, or friends.

## *Distance Learning*

To further enhance training opportunities for rural communities, three free web modules have been developed and are available on-line at www.ithaca.edu/aging/training and on CD-ROM. These are:

1. *Real Problems with Real Solutions: A Practice Approach to Geriatric Depression* Presenter: Lisa A. Kendall, MSW. This session explores common myths about depression in older adults, and addresses causes, symptoms, screening, diagnosis and treatment approaches.
2. *Safe at Home.* Presenter: Carol John, M.ED., OT. This session identifies ways in which older persons can be helped to age-in-place by enhancing their autonomy, reducing risk of harm through change of habits and the use of affordable products, and participating in meaningful activities.
3. *Practical Strategies to Reduce Falls.* Presenters: Katherine Beissner, PhD, PT and Terri Hoppenrath, MS, PT. This session reviews fall risk factors and modifications, how to administer basic tests that clarify fall risk, referral and evaluation, and the role of a physical therapist in reducing the risk of falls.

## *Assessment of the Model*

The County Community Team approach strengthens networks by involving participation of facilities and organizations who ordinarily may not communicate or collaborate. It also builds on shared training needs enabling expansion of training beyond that which is mandated. At the same time it enhances opportunities to expand the knowledge and skills of the broader health care/aging services workforce pool. Community training which targets frontline workers acknowledges the importance and value of their work and helps to enhance morale. Ultimately County Community Teams build capacity for continuing collaborative training events without the Geriatric Education Center (GEC) involvement.

## Summary

The development and implementation of successful and appropriate program responses to the needs of rural elders are constrained by myths that obscure the reality of aging in rural places. A lack of dollars, health and social service professionals, transportation, political clout, and understanding of rural diversity, serve as barriers to providing services to this population. Many rural elders lack access to appropriate community-based services that support independence and allow for consumer choice. Successful program approaches do exist, but little evaluation research has been conducted on their operation, and the training of professionals for rural practice is lacking. Flexibility, innovation, and public/private collaboration, have and will remain important ingredients to local responses to local needs. Federal and state agencies can serve rural elders best by providing more recognition of rural needs, more dollars, more flexibility, and more education/training resources.

## REFERENCES

Coward, R. T., DeWeaver, K. L., Schmidt, F. E., & Jackson, R. W. (1983). Mental health practice in rural environments: A frame of reference. *International Journal of Mental Health, 12*(1–2), 3–24.

Eberts, P. G. & Merschrod, K. (2003). *Socioeconomic trends and well-being indicators in New York State: 1950–2000.* Albany, NY: New York State Legislative Commission on Rural Resources.

Golant, S. (2003). The urban-rural distinction in gerontology. An update of research. In H. W. Whal, R. J. Scheidt, & P. G. Windley (Eds.). *Aging in context: Socio-physical environments. Annual Review of Gerontology and Geriatrics* (pp. 280–312). New York: Springer.

Krout, J. A. (1986). *The aged in rural America.* Westport, CT: Greenwood Press.

Krout, J. A. (1994a). *Providing community-based services to the rural elderly.* Thousand Oaks: Sage.

Krout, J. A. (1994b). *Area agencies on aging: A national longitudinal rural-urban comparison.* Final report to the AARP Andrus Foundation, Ithaca, NY: Ithaca College.

Krout, J. A. (1998). Services and service delivery in rural environments. In R. T. Coward & J. A. Krout, *Aging in rural settings* (pp. 247–266). New York: Springer.

Krout, J. A. (2003). Rural elders: Meeting their needs. R. J. Ham, R. T. Goins, & D. K. Brown (Eds.). *Best practices in service delivery to the rural elderly.* Morgantown, WV: West Virginia Center on Aging.

U.S. Census Bureau (2001). *Profiles of general demographic characteristics, 2000 Census of Population and Housing, United States.* Washington, DC: U.S. Government Printing Office.

*Chapter 6*

# Meeting the Rural Nursing Shortage Needs:
## An Evening/Weekend Nursing Program

### CLAIRE LIGEIKIS-CLAYTON

## Introduction

An evening/weekend nursing program (EWNP) at Broome Community College was developed to respond to the nursing shortage and to give individuals an opportunity to attend school while working full time. We unexpectedly found that the evening/weekend nursing program attracted a strong cohort of rural students. This discussion will focus on the nature of the EWNP, demographics of students enrolled, successes/shortcomings of the program and future directions.

### *Literature Search*

Evening/weekend nursing programs are not a new concept in nursing. However, the nursing literature is limited as to evaluation of EWNPs. Davis, Shiber, and Allen (1984) discussed the creation of a weekend program for registered nurses who worked full time and wished to receive their baccalaureate degrees. Findings revealed most students successfully completed the program and about half of them furthered their educations for advanced nursing degrees. O'Connor and Bevil (1996) reported outcomes of full time day and part time evening nursing students. Results included evening students working more and being older than their daytime cohorts. Evening students earned more As and experienced fewer failures. Donsky and Cox

(1994) cited research of Licensed Practical Nurses (LPNs) at Seminole Community College in Florida. Findings indicated that 62.2% were over 40 years of age, 51.2% worked 40 hours or more per week and 51.8% had interest in studying part time to become an RN. The reasons listed for not pursuing education were time, incongruent class hours and cost. Research conducted by Boyce (2000) concluded that students sought flexibility in course scheduling due to family and work responsibilities and desired programs that could be completed in three years or less. Karlowicz, Wiles, Bishop, and Lakin (2003), who surveyed Registered Nurse (RN) students enrolled and/or graduated in a weekend baccalaureate program, found strengths identified were the ability to work, small class size, faculty support and quality of instruction (p. 80). Limitations included feeling undervalued by faculty as weekend students vs. weekday students, inadequate clinicals on Saturdays and Sundays, and isolation from the larger campus (p. 80).

As we can see from the above findings, what students want in flexible nursing programs has not changed. Student demographics have not changed either. Based on these consistent findings, it is necessary for nursing programs to design creative curricula to support current health care workers and LPNs who desire to obtain their RN degrees.

## History of the Evening/Weekend Nursing Program at Broome Community College

Based on many anecdotal inquiries received by the department of nursing regarding part-time study and non-traditional course offerings, the nursing faculty considered an evening/weekend option. Current students in our daytime program were surveyed as to interest in a part time EWNP and the response was positive, more than 50% of approximately 135 students, for development of this option. Additionally, the Advisory Committee to the Nursing Department, whose members were nurse administrators of area health care facilities, reported that many of their employees could not attend school while working full time. Upgrading of current employees was an attractive option and employers were willing to pay for their employees' education. In reviewing the feasibility of an EWNP, the nursing department personnel also examined the success of a local LPN program, which was offered as an evening/weekend option and consistently had full enrollment. Another factor that was taken into consideration was the amount of inquiries from individuals who wished to make career changes or workers who had been displaced from their current positions.

Rather than expand our full time day program to meet the needs of the nursing shortage, an EWNP seemed a viable option. Additionally, with other nursing schools in the area, there was a shortage of clinical placements. The weekend clinical option did not overwhelm the current clinical sites.

Development of the evening/weekend nursing program began in Spring 2001. Input from existing students in the day program was sought as to scheduling options. Implementation began in Spring 2002.

## Design of the Evening/Weekend Nursing Program

The EWNP was designed to complete in three years or six semesters on a part time basis. (The day program is two years full time.) It assumes that students will enter the program with the required pre-requisites and liberal arts courses completed. Students take one nursing course, seven credits, each semester on a sequential basis. The nursing courses meet two evenings per week and every other weekend. The evening section includes didactic instruction and nursing laboratory sections that meet from 5 pm to 8 pm. There is open laboratory time before and after classes for students to practice their skills. Clinicals are offered every other weekend on Saturdays and Sundays during the day. These weekends remain constant throughout the semester since many of our students work the opposite weekends in health care facilities.

## Implementation

The EWNP was implemented in January 2002 with 20 students accepted into the program. In January 2003, enrollment was increased to 27 students due to a worsening nursing shortage and a long list of individuals awaiting acceptance into the program. Enrollment in January 2004 was 29 students.

## Methodology

A survey developed by the author included: (a) demographic information; (b) work status; (c) student status, part time vs. full time; (d) attraction into the EWNP; (e) study habits; and (f) satisfaction of resources. Surveying of existing students in the EWNP was conducted in Spring 2004. The survey was given to students in all three cohorts, during the 8th week of the semester. The cohorts were admitted in: (a) Spring 2002, (b) Spring 2003, and (c) Spring 2004. Of the 24 freshmen, 20 completed the survey while 11 of the 20 students taking senior courses completed the survey. Total response rate was 70%.

## Results

### Age

The age groups of the EWNP students ranged as follows: 29% were 20–29 years, 21% were 30–39 years, and 50% were 40–49 years. The ages of the EWNP students were mostly congruent with the day program however there was a slight increase in the 40–49 age group of the evening/weekend cohort.

### Gender

Females in the EWNP were 87% and males 13%. There were 3% more males in the EWNP compared to the day program.

### Ethnicity

Of the total evening/weekend program population, 94% of the students were white, 3% African American, and 3% Hispanic. The ethnicities of both the evening/weekend program and day programs were mostly congruent and mirrored the population of our region. However, approximately 3% of our day students were from Ukraine. In anecdotal inquiries with Ukrainian students, they cited the need to go to school full time for financial aid purposes and the desire to finish the degree in two years as reasons for not enrolling in the evening/weekend program.

## Full Time/Part Time Student Status

In the EWNP, 16% of the students were full time and 84% were part time. The day program had an opposite pattern with approximately 15% of the students being part time and 85% full time.

## Geographic Residence

Respondents reported that 29% lived in suburban areas, 17% in urban areas and 54% in rural areas. The largest group, 45%, of our EWNP students were from Binghamton, a city with a population of 47,380 in 2000. There were 38% from surrounding towns and 17% were from outlying areas over 25 miles away. Unfortunately, the day program was not analyzed for geographic residence. However, based on EWNP geographic residence only, these findings certainly have implications for future planning of alternative options in course offerings since 55% of the students report living out of the city limits of the college.

## Present Occupations

Respondents reported themselves as LPNs (35%) and in health related positions (60%). The remaining respondents were in unrelated positions (5%). These results show a higher percentage of LPNs in the EWNP than the day program. Since many of our LPN population work full time, these findings are indicative of the need for LPNs to attend RN study on a part time basis.

## Previous Education

Respondents who had previous education were LPNs (29%), Associate Degrees (35%) and Bachelor of Science (BS) Degrees (6%). Those with previous Associate Degrees identified their degrees in Physical Therapy Assistant, Medical Laboratory Technology, Health Information Technology, Medical Assistant, Business, English, and Criminal Justice. Individuals with a BS Degree identified their degrees in Political Science and Natural Sciences.

## Why the Evening/Weekend Nursing Program

When EWNP students were asked why they chose this option, 61% of the respondents stated "to upgrade position in health care," 42% "for job opportunities," 29% "for salary and benefits," and 19% "a complete change in careers."

## Study Time Outside the Classroom

Respondents were asked how much study time they spend outside the classroom per week including: (a) studying for exams, (b) reading, (c) preparation of lab, and (d) clinicals. Responses were as follows: (a) 0–10 hours per week, 17%; (b) 11–20 hours per week, 57%; (c) 21–30 hours per week, 23%; and (d) over 30 hours per week, 3%.

## Satisfaction with Resources

Resources evaluated by the respondents included Library, Nursing Skills Center Lab, Learning Assistance Center, and faculty availability. Findings included 35% of the respondents were not satisfied with available times in these facilities. However, 94% were satisfied with faculty availability. Ten percent of the respondents desired tapes and computer assisted instruction (CAI) on-line.

**Table 1**
*Retention of Students*

|  | Spring 2002 (n=20) | Spring 2003 (n=27) | Spring 2004 (n=29) |
|---|---|---|---|
| Withdrawals | 9 | 8 | 2 |
| Continuing Program | 8 | 5 | 27 |
| Transferred to Day Program | 2 | 8 | 0 * |
| Failures | 1 | 6 | 0 |
| Retention | 50% | 48% | 93% |

(* Transfer no longer an option in Spring 2004)

The above chart does not demonstrate high retention rates in the EWNP and is consistent with the daytime program. However, in exit interviews with the chairperson of the nursing department, the majority of students who withdrew did not do so for academic reasons, but for personal reasons. Anecdotally, this is different from the daytime program in which the majority of withdrawals are due to academic failure. The nursing faculty found that students in the EWNP who work full time had unrealistic expectations as to the amount of schoolwork outside the classroom. There is a similar unrealistic under expectation among the day-time students. Therefore the faculty developed a nursing documentary regarding success in nursing in which current and former students discussed the demands of the nursing program. We are hopeful that this documentary and the discussion of time management at registration will assist students in making better decisions regarding enrollment in nursing.

## Advantages of Evening/Weekend Program

The EWNP caters to students who have full time jobs and are unable to attend school in the traditional manner. Since many of the students in the EWNP are full time workers, they come to the educational arena with motivation and work ethics needed to be successful in school. We have therefore found a higher caliber of student in this program compared to our day program. Grade point averages (GPAs) reported by the respondents were: (a) 55% with 3.6–4.0, (b) 15% with 3.1–3.5 and (c) 30% with 2.5–3.0. Daytime students were not surveyed regarding their GPA.

Another advantage found is that the small classes inherent in the EWNP leads to more interaction between faculty and students. The average size of the day program for entering freshmen is 100 students versus 30 students in the EWNP.

A large population of our EWNP is the LPN. We have found that LPNs are very successful in our RN program and have a high graduation rate compared to generic students. The LPN has demonstrated success in nursing, has taken National Council Licensure Examination — Practical Nurse (NCLEX–PN), and has realistic expectations regarding the nursing profession. When nursing programs are looking at retention/graduation rates, the LPN becomes a desired student in RN programs.

Clinical sites on the weekend were at first thought to be a limitation but really became an advantage. Our program has access to most of the clinical facilities on the weekends and therefore we are able to provide students with excellent experiences. Students like two clinical days in a row because they can care for the same patients and be more involved in the continuum of care. We do have somewhat of a struggle placing students in community settings, but faculty have been very creative in scheduling different experiences. For example, if we cannot go to senior citizens centers on weekends, we use the local shopping mall.

The final advantage of the EWNP is our department is doing its part to ease the nursing shortage since we are now graduating more students from our program.

## Lessons Learned

Approval of the Evening/Weekend Nursing Program was dependant on our department being able to provide the same quality and consistency found in our day program. We therefore use full time faculty in both the day and evening programs. While faculty do not work overload, it has been difficult for them to teach in both programs. All full time faculty rotate teaching in the EWNP according to their areas of expertise. Our Department has also received an additional full time faculty line so that rotation in the EWNP is less. The nursing department has also received release time, three hours per semester, for an evening/weekend coordinator.

Staffing has been somewhat problematic for weekend clinicals. Most of our full time faculty do not teach clinicals on the weekends and therefore we rely on adjuncts. Communication between full time faculty and adjuncts is sometimes difficult. We are fortunate however that our adjuncts attend monthly faculty meetings so that consistent collaboration can occur.

We began our EWNP with the intent that students could switch tracks and go from the day program to the EWNP and vice versa. This proved problematic however and record keeping within the department became unwieldy. The option to switch programs was stopped in 2004.

## Future Directions

Our department has been pleased with the success of the EWNP. Our area health care facilities are equally pleased that there are more graduates and that their full time employees have an opportunity to advance careers.

A concern raised by the EWNP students is access to resources. We are investigating on-line availability of required CAI, videos, etc., so that students can access these resources from home. We are additionally working with support personnel such as the learning assistance center to expand evening services.

The EWNP has taught us that non-traditional course offerings are necessary to improve access to educational opportunities for individuals who wish to be educated yet are not the traditional student. Perhaps investigating the feasibility of putting nursing curricula on-line, especially for LPN students, needs to be explored more fully. Classroom and laboratory content could be put on line so that students would only need to attend laboratory skills demonstrations and clinical rotations. Perhaps partnering with outlying health care agencies to provide clinicals in students' home base would open access to rural areas of health care.

## Summary

There is a viable market for nursing students who wish to pursue RN studies while working full time. This market has a great cohort of LPNs who are unable to attend school in the traditional manner. Additionally, displaced workers from unrelated careers are attracted to RN programs because nursing is seen as a career in which demands will continue far into the future. Thinking outside the box is necessary if we wish to reach different populations and rural health care areas. Nursing programs are in a position to be the prime catalyst that corrects the nursing shortage today and tomorrow.

## REFERENCES

Boyce, B. (2000). *Development of a model for a part-time evening/weekend program at Lawrence Memorial/Regis College Collaborative Nursing Program with a plan for implementation and evaluation* (Doctoral dissertation, 2000). Florida: Nova Southeastern University.

Davis, A., Shiber, S., & Allen J. (1984). Weekend college. *Nursing Outlook, 32*(5), 259–261.

Donsky, A. & Cox, S. (1994). *The feasibility of an evening LPN to RN transition program.* Sanford, Florida: Seminole Community College Nursing Department (ERIC Document reproduction service, No. ED37589).

Karlowicz, K., Wiles, L., Bishop, J., & Lakin, M. (2003). The promise and perils of a weekend nursing program. *Nurse Educator, 28*(2), 77–82.

O'Connor, P., & Bevil C. (1996). Academic outcomes and stress in full-time day and part-time evening baccalaureate nursing students. *Journal of Nursing Education, 35,* 245–251.

*Chapter 7*

# Using the Concepts of the Nursing Paradigm to Sustain Rural Populations

### CAROLYN PIERCE

**Abstract:** Rural nurses are finding that the commonly used components of nursing's paradigm have taken on new meanings over time. As Kuhn theorized, a subspecialty may produce revolutionary changes in thinking that do not alter thinking in other subspecialties. The historical foundation of rural concepts and current findings from rural research are utilized to describe the nursing paradigm through a different lens. Two important threads connecting the rural nursing paradigm include vulnerability and resilience.

## Introduction

Kuhn (1996) wrote that a paradigm may serve many groups, but that it may not necessarily be utilized in the same way for all members. Subspecialties, according to Kuhn, may produce revolutions in thinking that do not affect other subspecialties in a similar fashion. It would appear that rural nursing is experiencing revolutionary changes in its paradigm. These changes are the result of over 25 years of attention to the unique nature of rural nursing. Long and Weinert (1989) set the tone for attention to the concepts of work and health beliefs, isolation and distance, self reliance, lack of anonymity, outsider/insider, and oldtimer/newcomer in rural populations. Soon thereafter, Bushy (1991a, 1991b) edited two books focused on rural nursing, in which the authors highlighted vulnerable populations and issues related to nursing and health care delivery in rural places.

Since that time, rural nursing has received increasing attention. Currently, many nursing researchers are actively working in rural settings all over the world. A rural nursing textbook (Bushy,

2000) and several other rural nursing books are available. *The Online Journal of Rural Health and Nursing* provides access to research about rural nursing, and many nursing and health care journals address rural health care issues. Nurses are active collaborators with other health care disciplines to improve rural health. The Rural Nurse Organization (RNO) promotes collaboration and education of rural nurses. Many universities offer courses in undergraduate and graduate courses in rural nursing. One PhD program in rural nursing is located at Binghamton University in upstate New York.

The results of this subspecialty's body of work show evidence that the basic concepts of nursing's paradigm of human being, environment, health and nursing (Fawcett, 2005), reflect a different view from those used by the nursing profession as a whole. This discussion will describe the current state of these concepts as found in the extant rural nursing literature.

## *Human Beings*

The concept of human beings, according to Fawcett (2005) "refers to the individuals, if individuals are recognized in a culture, as well as to the families, communities, and other groups or aggregates who are participants in nursing" (p. 6). While rural nurses would generally concur with this definition, there is evidence that rural dwellers have uniquely significant and complex attributes that cannot be ignored. Because rural areas are vastly different geographically and culturally, and because many rural demographics are changing at a rapid rate, there is great difficulty in accurately characterizing rural dwellers. About 48 million people lived in 2,052 rural counties in the United States according to the 2000 census, increasing 10% since the 1990 census (National Advisory Committee on Rural Health and Human Services, 2004, p. 4). Rural dwelling is associated with poorer health outcomes for all age groups and for more chronic diseases in the older population than is found in urban counterparts (Glasgow, Johnson, & Morton, 2004). Rural mental health issues appear to be different than in urban areas and include increasing methamphetamine use in teenagers and higher suicide rates in men (Lorenz, Wickrama, & Yeh, 2004).

Along with the differing health concerns are those uniquely rural attributes described in rural nursing literature. Bushy (2000) listed several recurring dimensions central to the concept of the rural person including: diversity, multicultural population, familiarity among locals, preference for care by a known person, and the dichotomy between newcomer (outsider) and oldtimer (insider) (p. 35). Bushy also addressed the issues of self-reliance and independence in health care decisions and the sense of hardiness that are often attributed to rural dwellers.

Additional factors have also been identified among rural dwellers when accessing health care. Horner et al. (1994) found that rural persons often waited before seeking healthcare because of limited financial resources, prior experiences with the health care system, and/or the belief that self-care was effective. If self-care was found to be ineffective, rural dwellers then evaluated their resources and tried to access the care they believed they needed. Tripp-Reimer (1982) alerted health care providers of the dichotomy that existed between analysis of the actions to obtain health care by Appalachian people and non-Appalachian caregivers. The potential clash of cultures may contribute significantly to reliance of rural dwellers upon lay care rather then entering into the mainstream but somewhat daunting health care system.

Long and Weinert (1989) found that the ability to work, a prominent attribute of rural dwellers, also involves feelings of self-reliance and independence. These factors embody the strong desire found in many rural dwellers to do for one's self. For example, elderly rural women with higher levels of independence were found to have increased feelings of self-confidence and self-competence (Chafey, Sullivan, & Shannon, 1998). The sense of self-reliance may also be in play when rural dwellers forgo traditional health care facilities to seek health care or advice from family members and lay health providers.

Rural dwellers often describe feelings of pride in their sense of hardiness (Bigbee, 1991). Hardiness has been described as a moderating or buffering factor on stress, which then impacts the perception of illness and is reflected in efforts regarding health promotion, independence, self-reliance, and self-care. Hardiness entails three components including the interrelated concepts of challenge, control, and commitment (Bigbee, 1991). Within this conceptualization, challenge is conceived as the response to the complexities of life which provide opportunities for growth, flexibility and openness. Persons with an internal locus of control are thought to be more likely to feel that their actions will alter or modify stress into positive challenges. A sense of commitment provides a meaningful sense of purpose within their environment. The interrelatedness of these concepts gives rise to health promoting responses to the stress inherent in daily life.

Resistance of rural dwellers to outsider interventions as described by Long and Weinert (1989) is an area of concern for rural nurses. Bushy (2000) described a resistance to outside bureaucratic influence in health care that must be accounted for, since many rural health care facilities have a formal interface with hospital systems from outside the area. Health care providers in these systems may not be aware of local customs and norms influencing health care decisions. It has also been seen that rural dwellers may prefer to receive health care from persons that they know who live in the community (Bushy, 2000). However, such close-knit relationships can lead to problems with the lack of confidentiality regarding health care in rural communities (Long & Weinert, 1989).

## *Environment*

Environment, according to Fawcett (2005), is comprised of the significant others, the physical environment, and the environment where nursing occurs, entailing the local, regional, national, and worldwide cultural, social, political, and economic conditions that impact the person's health. Clearly the environment has the potential to have a much broader impact on health care in rural settings. Bushy (2000) cited three dominant and interrelated dimensions of ruralness including occupational, ecological, and sociocultural dimensions. The occupational dimension goes beyond agriculture to include any labor of primary production and the support services for those industries. The ecological dimension refers to the spatial relationship with the surroundings. The sociocultural dimension includes those relationships with family and neighbors as well as those with formal agencies. These relationships are heavily influenced by the cultural norms of the area and can vary widely from place to place.

The term rural dweller is often associated with a feeling of connection with the land, and this is especially true for those persons whose livelihood is directly related to such industries as crops, logging, fishing and hunting, and recreations. Authors de la Rue and Coulson (2003) described findings of research with rural women who felt a spatial relationship to their surrounding because they were "living on the land" (p. 192). Rural dwellers may also describe that they prefer the slower pace, less pollution, and the geography of the area that gives them strength (Pierce, 2001). Similarly, Thurston and Meadows (2003) reported symbols associated with rural life by middle aged rural dwelling women to be clean air, no hustle and bustle, the presence of wild life, the freedom to have domestic animals, the beauty of nature, open spaces, and knowing people who live nearby. They also found rural life to be health-enhancing.

However, it is also true that the realities of the rural environment extend beyond the idyllic notions many persons hold about rural life to include harsh and sometimes dangerous surroundings. While only one-third of all motor vehicle crashes occur in rural areas, over two-thirds of deaths from these accidents occur in rural areas (National Rural Health Association [NRHA], n.d.). Rural dwellers are nearly two times more likely to die from unintentional injuries than urban dwellers, and are at a much higher risk of death from gunshot wounds (NRHA, n.d.). Widespread abuse of alcohol by rural teens may contribute to this problem.

## *Health*

According to Fawcett (2005), health is "the human processes of living and dying" (p. 6). There is a substantive body of knowledge supporting the premise that health is defined by rural persons as the ability to work or to do normal daily activities (Weinert & Long, 1987; Weinert & Long, 1991; Pierce, 2001). Lee and Winters (2004) noted that this definition has changed somewhat to include being able to function and to "do the things you want to do and feel good at it, both working and playing" (p. 7). The authors related this to differences in populations or to changing attitudes over time.

In one study older widowed women thought that health was not being ill or having sickness complaints (de la Rue & Coulson, 2003). The women also felt that they needed to maintain their health in order to continue living on the land in rural areas. Similarly, Thurston and Meadows (2003) found that living in rural areas was not seen as a threat to health by middle-aged women, but noted that this perception may be seen differently by women who have small children or who no longer are capable of driving a distance for health care.

## *Nursing*

Fawcett (2005) defined nursing as "the actions taken by nurses on behalf of or in conjunction with the person, and the goals or outcomes of nursing actions" (p. 6). Rural nursing has been defined by Long and Weinert (1989) as the "provision of health care by professional nurses to persons living in sparsely populated areas" (p. 122). Scharff (1998) wrote that rural nurses must be able to function within the fluid intersection between nursing and other professional disciplines. This practice requires a wide range and depth of practice knowledge and ability, while dealing with overlapping clinical areas. While providing nursing in rural settings, nurses must balance the generalist with a wide range of specific skills. Rural nurses are often called upon to function outside of the traditional nursing role and must navigate the issues of role diffusion (Long & Weinert, 1989). In hospital settings those intersections with other disciplines may mean that nurses are performing functions normally under the responsibility of other health care professionals such as pharmacists and physicians, as well as laboratory and diagnostic personnel. In isolated homes and communities the level of role diffusion may be even greater.

Nurses in rural areas must understand the unique complexity of the rural experience. They must understand the unique conceptions of health and illness of rural dwellers. For instance, nurses who practice in rural areas need to understand that rural dwellers may delay treatment due to the need to work, or only attend health care appointments that fit into their work schedules. They also may find that rural dwellers delay treatment due to reliance on self-care or treatment from insiders. The lack of trust of outsiders may be ameliorated by nurses who enter into activities in the community in order to increase personal acceptance. They must be aware that this process of acceptance may take a considerable length of time (Long & Weinert, 1989). In addition, health care providers often must be willing to take a relatively long period of time to get to know rural persons while trust is established (e.g., the insider/outsider issue) and must factor adequate time to establish rapport and trust into the process of health care provision. Seasoned rural nurses also know that they must not hurry or appear to be rushed for time

Rural nurses often know their clients in a number of everyday roles including neighbor or relative, and through organizations such as churches or school activities. They may find that they are called upon to be a nurse outside of their work environment, and have a sense of "always being on duty" (Weinert & Long, 1991). The positive aspect of this knowledge is that rural nurses know their clients in their routine lives, and thus may be able to anticipate health problems, know personal and family histories, work situation, diet, substance use/abuse, pressing needs at home that may prevent obtaining necessary health care, financial concerns, etc. Rural nurses also tend to know what health care services are available locally.

## *Vulnerability/Resilience*

A thread that weaves throughout the concepts of the rural paradigm is that of vulnerability and resiliency in the rural population. Vulnerable populations, according to Flaskerud and Winslow (1998, p. 69) are social groups with increased susceptibility or risk of negative health outcomes. Individuals as well as populations can experience vulnerability (de Chesnay, 2005). Groups that have been considered vulnerable include high-risk mothers and infants, chronically ill and the disabled, persons living with HIV/AIDS, the mentally ill and disabled, alcohol and substance abusers, suicide and homicide prone behaviors, abusive families, homeless persons, and immigrants and refugees (de Chesnay, 2005).

Leight (2003) listed indicators of vulnerability that are often attributed to rural dwellers including poverty, loss of jobs, level of education, homelessness, distance to health care, inadequate health care resources, less than optimal nutrition, exercise, and sleep, less likely to use seat belts, have pap smears, get immunizations, and have dental and physical examinations, increased motor vehicle accidents and accidental work-related injuries, increased chronic illness, and infant mortality. Because many of these issues are experienced by rural dwellers and some may have multiples issues, vulnerability may be compounded. In addition, the potential for lack of screening and/or treatment services leads to further risk of alterations in health.

Flaskerud and Winslow (1998) proposed a conceptual framework of vulnerable populations that relates resource availability, relative risk, and health status of the community as measured by morbidity and mortality. As societal and environmental resources are limited, relative risk for poor health rises and contributes to increased morbidity and mortality. Increased morbidity leads to decreased resource availability. Each of these factors has unique applications in rural settings.

Vulnerability related to environment is intensified by distance to health care services if they are available, lack of transportation, and in some climates to weather related obstacles. While some authors have not found distance to be a factor in seeking healthcare (Pierce, 2001; Thurston & Meadows, 2003), availability of transportation to traverse that distance does have an impact on utilization of health care services. In rural North Carolina, persons with a driver's license or family or friends who drove them were significantly more likely to make regular and chronic care visits (Arcury, Preisser, Gesler, & Powers, 2005). Because public transportation in rural areas is a rarity, rural dwellers without access to personal transportation may be unable to receive both acute and chronic care.

Vulnerability related to how health is defined by rural dwellers difference in the definition of health as well as expectations for health care services. Rural Virginians were found to "make do" or adjust to what services were available in their communities (Huttlinger, Schaller-Ayers, Lawson, & Ayers, 2003). While they saw the importance of obtaining health care to maintain health, they felt it was difficult to obtain. Respondents felt that because they lived in poor areas that they expected poor health care as well. Thurston and Meadows (2003) warned health care providers that viewing a rural area as an unhealthy place may be at odds with how the area is viewed by residents. Thus the lack of congruity may lead to communication breakdown and a further detrimental effect on health care provision.

Vulnerability related to nursing care can be seen on several levels. While the impending shortage of nurses in America and internationally is well documented, the shortage of rural nurses has distinct issues that may ultimately have serious ramifications in rural areas. The nursing shortage can be anticipated to be more severe in frontier and rural areas because (a) frontier and rural providers have less economic resources to compete with urban providers, (b) most nurses were not prepared educationally to work in non-urban settings, and (c) frontier and rural communities depend on non-hospital care more than the urban counterparts (Frontier Education Center [FEC], 2004). At the present time, more than 50% of frontier counties with hospitals have a shortage of nurses (FEC, 2004). This can only be expected to worsen. The shortage is not only felt in rural hospitals, but is especially acute in school nursing programs and in home health agencies.

Recruiting for nursing positions in some rural areas can take 60% longer than in non-rural areas (FEC, 2004). When nurses can be recruited, they do not always have the necessary skills for the position. Most nurses in rural areas have an associate degree and thus are not prepared for the increased independent responsibilities necessary in changing health care systems. Further, rural nurses are often unable to find access to higher education because of their daily commitments and the distance to educational facilities. Mahnken (2001, p. 5) identified "barriers to continuing nursing education." These included "the isolating nature of distance education, lack of support and culture of learning in employing institutions, cost to the individual and family, lack of professional recognition and career structure, professional isolation, and competition for time with family" and work commitments (p. 5). Nurses in rural areas need a broad knowledge and skill base as well as an increased level of independence and a strong sense of self-reliance (Britten, Hahn, & Ragusa, 2003). It is critical that rural nurses have not only didactic educational content on rural nursing but clinical experience in rural areas as well.

Caregivers of vulnerable populations can develop methods to promote resilience in vulnerable populations (de Chesnay, Wharton, & Pamp, 2005). Resilience is the "capacity for transcending obstacles, which is present to some degree in all human beings" (de Chesnay et al., 2005, p. 31). Rural dwellers have long been considered a resilient group. Leipert and Reutter (2005) theorized that rural women developed resilience through strategies of becoming hardy, making the best of the situation, and supplementing what the area had to offer (p. 56).

Resilience may be augmented by the rural environment. Rural living was found to contribute to the sense of wholeness as well as a spiritual underpinning for older rural women in New South Wales (de la Rue & Coulson, 2003). Strong ties to the geographical area and the sense of community and to people who have lived there for generations lead to a feeling of allegiance and pride (Huttlinger et al., 2003). Thus, neighbors were considered family even if blood relationships were not present, as community members are known to watch out for and support neighbors in need.

Resilience in health can be augmented by the strength found in the rural life. Rural women have been reported to hold a holistic view of health including physical, mental, spiritual, and social aspects (Thurston & Meadows, 2003). Rural life has been ascribed with life-enhancing qualities.

Resilience related to nursing may be enhanced through the strength of relationships between clients and nurses who are familiar with each other in multiple roles in the community. Nurses who live in the community know the burdens of the area as well as historical and political factors that are important to providing comprehensive care. One way nurses can augment resilience is by spending quality time with the client. This need for quality time with primary providers is thought to be related to a strong sense of community and the need to bring outsiders into the community (Huttlinger et al., 2003). Nurses can also focus on supporting self-management of health care. Intrapersonal factors such as assertiveness, coping behaviors, knowledge, and self-efficacy are key in engaging in therapeutic behaviors and accessing social supports to improve health and quality of life (Dorsey & Murdaugh, 2003) particularly in rural populations.

# Conclusion

Many nurses question whether rural nursing is a distinct specialty (Brown-Schott, Britten, & Walker, 2003; Bushy, 2000; Scharff, 1998; Weinert & Long, 1991). As this issue is debated, the basic tenets of the paradigm must be closely scrutinized. Attention to changing meanings and context are critical. Rural nurses face multiple challenges, including limited resources and clients who generally are more vulnerable to poorer health outcomes than their urban counterparts. However, they also have valuable inside knowledge about their clients, many of whom have great capacity to shoulder adversity and develop resiliency. Rural nurses are learning about the many attributes of rural life that can alter the prevailing wisdom about how they think about nursing actions and responsibilities. These insights will provide invaluable guidance to other rural nurses, and to their nursing counterparts in non-rural settings as well.

## REFERENCES

Arcury, T., Preisser, J., Gesler, W., & Powers, J. (2005). Access to transportation and health care utilization in a rural region. *The Journal of Rural Health, 21,* 31–38.

Bigbee, J. (1991). The concept of hardiness as applied to rural nursing. In A. Bushy (Ed.), *Rural Nursing* (Vol. 1) (pp. 39–58). Newbury Park: Sage.

Britten, M., Hahn, L., & Ragusa, T. (2003). Teaching rural nursing to urban students. In. M. Collins, (Ed.), *Teaching/learning activities for rural community-based nursing practice* (pp. 54–71). Binghamton, NY: Binghamton University.

Brown-Schott, N., Britten, M., & Walker, K. (2003). Rural nursing curriculum development. *Teaching/learning activities for rural community-based nursing practice* (pp. 13–33). Binghamton, NY: Binghamton University.

Bushy, A. (2000). *Orientation to nursing in the rural community.* Thousand Oaks: Sage.

Bushy, A. (1991a). *Rural nursing: Volume 1.* Newbury Park: Sage.

Bushy, A. (1991b). *Rural nursing: Volume 2.* Newbury Park: Sage

Chafey, K., Sullivan, T., & Shannon, A. (1998). Self-reliance: Characterization of their own autonomy by elderly rural women. In H. Lee, (Ed.), *Conceptual basis for rural nursing* (pp. 156–177). New York: Springer.

de Chesnay, M. (Ed.). (2005). Vulnerable populations: Vulnerable people. *Caring for the vulnerable: Perspectives in nursing theory, practice, and research* (pp. 3–12). Sudbury: Jones & Bartlett.

de Chesnay, M., Wharton, R., & Pamp, C. (2005). Cultural competence, resilience, & advocacy. In M. de Chesnay (Ed.), *Caring for the vulnerable: Perspectives in nursing theory, practice, & research* (pp. 31–41). Sudbury, MA: Jones & Bartlett.

de la Rue, M. & Coulson, I. (2003). The meaning of health and well being: Voices from older women. *Rural and Remote Health 3 (Online),* Available: http://rrh.deakin.edu.au

Dorsey, C., & Murdaugh, C. (2003). The theory of self-care management for vulnerable populations. *Journal of Theory Construction and Testing, 7*(2), 43–47.

Fawcett, J. (2005). *Contemporary nursing knowledge: Analysis and evaluation of nursing models and theories,* (2nd ed.). Philadelphia: Davis.

Flaskerud, J., & Winslow, B. (1998). Conceptualizing vulnerable populations health-related research. *Nursing Research, 47*(2), 69–78.

Frontier Education Center. (2004). *Addressing the nursing shortage: Impacts and innovations in frontier America.* Ojo Sarco, NM: Author.

Glasgow, N., Johnson, L., & Morton, L. (2004). Introduction. In N. Glasgow, L. Morton, & N. Johnson, (Eds.), *Critical issues in rural health* (pp. 3–11). Ames, IA: Blackwell.

Horner, S., Ambrogne, J., Hanson, C., Hodnicki, D., Lopez, S., & Talmadge, C. (1994). Traveling for care: Factors influencing health care access for rural dwellers. *Public Health Nursing, 11*(3), 145–149.

Huttlinger, K., Schaller-Ayers, J., Lawson, T., & Ayers, J. (2003). Suffering it out: Meeting the needs of health care delivery in a rural area. *Online Journal of*

*Rural Nursing and Health Care*, 3(2), [Online]. Available: http://www.rno.org/journal/issues/Vol-3/issue-2/Huttlinger_article.htm

Kuhn, T. (1996). *The structure of scientific revolutions*, (3rd ed.). Chicago: University of Chicago Press.

Lee, H., & Winters, C. (2004). Testing nursing theory: Perceptions and needs of service providers. *Online Journal of Rural Nursing and Health*, 4(1), [Online]. Available: http://www.rno.org/journal/issues/Vol-4/issue-1/Lee_article.htm

Leight, S. (2003). Application of a vulnerable populations conceptual model to rural health. *Public Health Nursing*, 20, 440–448.

Leipert, B., & Reutter, L. (2005). Developing resilience: How women maintain their health in northern geographically isolated settings. *Qualitative Health Research*, 15(1), 49–65.

Long, K., & Weinert, C. (1989). Rural nursing: Developing the theory base. *Scholarly Inquiry for Nursing Practice: An International Journal*, 3, 113–127.

Lorenz, F., Wickrama, K., & Yeh, H. (2004). Rural mental health: Comparing differences and modeling change. In N. Glasgow, L. Morton, & N. Johnson, (Eds.), *Critical Issues in Rural Health* (pp. 75–88). Ames, IA: Blackwell.

Mahnken, J. (2001). Rural nursing and health care reforms: Building a social model of health. *Rural and Remote Health*, 104, 1–4.

National Advisory Committee on Rural Health and Human Services. (2004). The 2004 report to the secretary: Rural health and human service issues. Rockville, MD: Author.

National Rural Health Association, (n.d.). *What's different about rural health care?* Kansas City: MO. Author. Retrieved 2005 from http://www.nrharural.org/about/sub/different.html

Pierce, C. (2001). The impact of culture in rural women's descriptions of health. *The Journal of Multicultural Health and Nursing*, 7(1), 50–53, 56.

Scharff, J. (1998). The distinctive nature and scope of rural nursing practice: Philosophical issues. In H. Lee (Ed.), *Conceptual Basis for Rural Nursing* (pp. 19–38). New York: Springer.

Thurston, W. & Meadows, L. (2003). Rurality and health: Perspectives of rural mid-life women. *Rural and Remote Health*, 3(3), 219.

Tripp-Reimer, T. (1982). Barriers to health care: Variations in interpretation of Appalachian client behavior by Appalachian and non-Appalachian health professionals. *Western Journal of Nursing Research*, 4, 179–191.

Weinert, C., & Long, K. (1987). Understanding the health care needs of rural families. *Family Relations*, 36, 450–455.

Weinert, C., & Long, K. (1991). The theory and research base for rural nursing practice. In A. Bushy (Ed.), *Rural Nursing: Volume 1* (pp. 21–38). Newbury Park: Sage.

*Chapter 8*

# Quality of Life in Rural Women with Heart Failure: The State of the Science

CAROLYN PIERCE

## Introduction

*Rural Health: A Vision of 2010*, authored by the Federal Office of Rural Health Policy and the National Rural Health Association (1998), illustrates the quest for a rural America in which all persons have optimal health. Quality of life (QOL) has often been considered an important component of optimal health. QOL, or health-related quality of life (HRQOL) has a wide range of conceptual and operational definitions and in many respects remains a rather nebulous concept. Because of the lack of consensus about what constitutes QOL or HRQOL, it is critical that conceptual, cultural, and measurement issues be carefully considered when performing research in these areas.

A clear and succinct definition of QOL is difficult to discern because over the years this term has been used interchangeably with such concepts as functional status or capacity, well-being, and general health status (Haas, 1999). Indeed, some researchers question if QOL is really perceived health (Moons, 2004). Quality of survival assessments used after clinical trials or therapeutic interventions also include measures of functional status and subjective attitudes of the patient (Prutkin & Feinstein, 2002). Imprecision of the term health in our society also contributes to confusion about what this term signifies. QOL has been used to represent such widely divergent dimensions as emotional function, level of well-being, life satisfaction, happiness, intellectual level, social activity, financial status and employment, and level of symptoms including pain, nausea and vomiting, and fatigue (Prutkin & Feinstein, 2002).

Various professions bring divergent perspectives into the definition of QOL. For example, philosophers focus on the nature of human existence and the good life, ethicists consider social utility, and economist focus on allocation of resources. Physicians consider health and illness variables while nurses take a broader, holistic perspective of the person (Anderson & Burckhardt, 1999).

It is estimated that there may be 800 dimensions represented in the construct of QOL (Chung, Killingworth, & Nolan, 1997). Indeed this lack of precision about what QOL entails is further muddied by the plethora of tools used to assess QOL. Nearly 500 tools used to assess QOL are listed in the Patient-reported Outcome and Quality of Life Instruments Database (PROQOLID) (Mapi Research Trust, 2004). Over 800 QOL tools are indexed in the Online Guide to QOL Instruments (OGLA) (2005).

Chung, Killingworth, and Nolan (1997) suggested that even if there were consensus about the definition of QOL, it still may not be reasonable to assume that it is possible to understand or quantify the metaphysical structures of QOL. Because the ability to understand another person is based on humanly derived words, it may be impossible to reach a perfect understanding of such a subjective concept. The attempts to understand another persons' meaning using imprecise words can provide only an update of this partial understanding.

However, if the assumption is made that QOL can be studied and measured, careful consideration must be made of the conceptual and operational definitions of QOL and then in choosing a method of research that supports those definitions. This discussion will examine the current state of the science of QOL assessment as it pertains to rural women with heart failure.

## Why Measure QOL or HRQOL?

Research has shown that HRQOL is a significant predictor of HF-related hospitalization and mortality for persons with HF when compared to traditional clinical indicators (Chin & Goldman, 1998; Konstram et al., 1995; Stull, Clough, & Van Dussen, 2001). QOL also has been found to be important enough by some patients that they are willing to take medications that improve QOL but may also put them at increased risk of death (Rector et al., 1995).

The Agency for Health Care Policy and Research (now known as the Agency for Healthcare Research and Quality) developed guidelines for the treatment of HF (Konstram et al., 1995). These guidelines point to outcome measures beyond the traditional biologic markers to broader issues including HRQOL and decreasing mortality.

## Historical Evolution of QOL/HRQOL

The construct of QOL can be traced to the functional status tools developed by physicians in the mid part of the last century. One such tool, the Karnofsky Performance Scale, assessed the ability of cancer patients to perform normal activities as well as their need for medical care (Karnofsky & Burchenal, 1949). A similar tool developed by Katz, Ford, Moskowitz, Jackson, and Jaffe (1963) as an Index of Independence of Activities of Daily Living Scale was utilized for patients with hip fractures and chronic diseases to assess the patient's ability to perform such activities as bathing, dressing, toileting, transferring, feeding, and the level of continence. In 1969, Lawton and Brody developed the Activities of Daily Living Scale which addressed daily activities such as shopping, food preparation, housekeeping, laundry, use of the telephone, mode of transportation, responsibility for medications, and ability to handle finances. These tools were focused on a limited number of domains and utilized rating scales that were assessed by an outside observer.

Contemporaneous to the development of functional assessment tools, sociologists became interested in eliciting information about the effects of diseases and treatments from the patient's perspective. After the World Health Organization (WHO) described health as "a state of complete physical, mental, and social well-being and not merely the absence of disease or infirmity" (WHO, 1948, p. 100), clinicians became increasingly interested in measuring the subjective experience of health and illness along with more objective data because of increasing thought that life was more than a corporeal state and was influenced by environmental and social factors (Prutkin & Feinstein, 2002). Use of a normal life approach, as used in functional assessments, was seen to reveal quite different information than the use of an evaluative approach, such as an alteration in life satisfaction related to the impact of symptoms (Kaplan, 1988). Increasing attention to QOL in every day life was also reflected in the report from the Eisenhower Commission on National Goals that further elevated the issue of QOL as an area for concern for every American (President's Commission of National Goals: Goals for America, 1960).

Over time questions were raised about the appropriateness of QOL to provide information about the impact of symptoms and treatments on usual daily activities and well-being. It was thought that QOL was too global and that focusing on health aspects of the dimensions of QOL would allow for more precision. Thus, QOL was further delineated as HRQOL to assess the "impact of life conditions on function" (Kaplan, 1988, p. 382). Assessment of HRQOL often includes such domains as physical measures, behavior, and symptoms or feelings about health (Al-Kaade & Hauptman, 2001). Measures of HRQOL may focus on a broad subjective evaluation of well-being or on the subjective appraisal of life satisfaction (Kaplan, 1988).

## Culture and QOL

Culture has been found to impact perceptions and interpretations of illness, the meaning given to symptoms, the experience of the illness, and illness behaviors (Staniszewska, Ahmed, & Jenkinson, 1999). When using QOL measurement tools outside of the dominant American middle class, construct validity may be challenged (Maramaldi, Berkman, & Barusch, 2005). Administration to vulnerable populations including immigrants, people of different races, gay and lesbian people, and people with chronic illness or disabilities must be carefully considered. When assessing the impact of diseases or illness on HRQOL, understanding the differences in physiology between various cultural groups is critical (Staniszewska, Ahmed, & Jenkinson, 1999).

Corless, Nicholas, and Nokes (2001) outlined several concerns when adapting or translating QOL measures. A primary consideration is how the concept is perceived in the group in question as opposed to the norming population. Issues such as age, gender, sexual orientation, race, ethnicity, religion, education, and occupation must be considered in relationship to their impact on validity and reliability. Cultural diversity in a country must also be considered. For example, in a nation such as the U.S. where there are wide variations in culture vary from countries with a more homogenous population. Relevance of the concept must meet the concern of the population to be studied. For example, QOL may not be salient in an area where people are only concerned with survival. The conceptual equivalence across languages may not be comparable and thus some issues may need to be added or removed. The hegemony of the dominant American middle class which provide the norms for the majority of QOL instruments cannot be ignored.

## Conceptual Issues in Measurement of QOL

QOL can be considered as both a unidimensional and a multidimensional construct with most of the current literature favoring the later. Examples of unidimensional tools are those purely measuring physical function as previously described. Conversely, Haas (1999) defined QOL in part as "a multidimensional evaluation of an individual's current circumstances in the context of the culture and value systems in which they live and the values they hold. QOL is primarily a subjective sense of well-being encompassing physical, psychological, social and spiritual dimensions" (p. 219). An example of a multidimensional approach was used in a study of older women with HF by Janz et al. (2001). The authors used Wilson and Cleary's conceptual model of Patient Outcomes to test QOL and included the following dimensions: biological, symptom status, functional status, general health perception, overall QOL, value preferences, and social and psychological support.

If a multidimensional approach is chosen, there are two traditional methods to performing QOL assessment including psychometric evaluation and decision theory (Kaplan, 1988). Psychometric assessments provide separate scores for each of the dimensions chosen to represent QOL. An example of this is the Sickness Impact Profile (SIP) (Bergner, Bobbitt, Carter, & Gilson, 1981) which is a 136-item test with 12 scores. Conversely, decision theory provides a summary of weighted measures of QOL dimensions in a single score of QOL integrating various dimensions such as subjective function levels, morbidity and mortality. For example, many studies of medical interventions assess quality-adjusted life years (QALY) which are computed to integrate morbidity and mortality as an expression of health status in equivalents of well years of life (Kaplan, 1988). These measures are then used to discern cost effectiveness and/or cost utility. While increasing life expectancy is usually the desired outcome, considerations of the side effects of treatments must be factored in as well. For example, certain high blood pressure medications may increase longevity but may have serious side effects that the patient may find untenable (Kaplan, 1988).

While there is consensus that QOL is a multidimensional construct, there is a lack of consensus about the need to have multidimensional measures (Kaplan, 1988). A unidimensional approach is often used to assess QOL with a single question by asking a question such as "How do you rate your health?" using a Likert scale from "very good" to "very bad." Another strategy is use of a visual analog scale that allows the patient to mark how they assess their current health state on a 10-cm line with 0 corresponding to death, and 1 corresponding with perfect health. This mark is converted to numerical form by measuring the segment of the line from the 0 point to the mark and then dividing that by the total length of the line (Havranek et al., 2001).

QOL or HRQOL tools may be comprehensive or designed to be disease- or situation-specific (Kaplan, 1988). Commonly used comprehensive QOL or HRQOL instruments include the Medical Outcomes Study (MOS) Short Form (SF) 36, the Sickness Impact Profile (SIP) and the EQ-5D. The SF36 (Ware & Sherbourne, 1992) is a tool designed to measure health status. The EQ-5D (EuroQol, n.d.) is designed as a measure of health outcomes using the dimensions of mobility, self-care, usual activities, pain/discomfort, and anxiety/depression. These dimensions are graded in three levels including: no problem, some or moderate problem, and extreme problem. An accompanying visual analog scale can be used to measure self-rated health status. This tool has been designed to be self-administered, telephone administered, or used in a personal interview.

Two commonly used disease-specific tools for measurement of HRQOL for persons with HF include: the Minnesota Living with Heart Failure (LHFQ) Questionnaire and the Chronic Heart Failure Questionnaire (CHQ). The LHFQ (Rector & Cohn, 1992) was designed as a patient outcome questionnaire for use with medical interventions for patients with HF. This self-assessment tool covers two dimensions including physical and emotional on a Likert scale from no impact to high impact. The CHQ (Guyatt, Feeny, & Patrick, 1993) is a 16-item tool developed to measure subjective health status of persons with HF. Dimensions of the CHQ include dyspnea during daily activities, fatigue, emotional function. This tool is designed to be administered by a skilled observer. The New York Heart Association (NYHA) classification tool is frequently utilized in conjunction with other tools of physical assessment in studies of QOL in patients with HF and has been found to be major correlate of HRQOL in persons with HF (Westlake et al., 2002).

## Measurement of QOL in Patients with Heart Failure

Research has found that many studies of cardiac interventions about QOL do not define QOL or the designate the dimensions of QOL to be studied (Gill & Feinstein, 1994; Kinney, Burfitt, Stullenberger, Rees, & DeBolt, 1996). Without this information, it is impossible to assess if the measures used are appropriate. Indeed, many studies of QOL address interventions for the physiological dimensions and ignore the broader issues tested in multidimensional instruments (Anderson & Burckhardt, 1999; Kinney et al., 1996).

QOL instruments must meet the accepted norms for reliability, validity, and responsiveness. Decisions about the relative weighting of dimensions, timing of administration, frequency of administration, and the method of administration are equally critical (Al-Kaade & Hauptman, 2001). The authors also raise the question about the relationship of findings of the perceptions of health of the individual. They comment that "how much key physiologic measure have to change before there is an effect on perceived health or on the ability of a patient to live his/her life is not known" (Al-Kaade & Hauptman, 2001, p. 196).

The timing of testing of QOL in HF can be a at issue due to rapidly declining physical function, and/or increasing anxiety and even depression as the disease progresses (vanJaarsveld, Sanderman, Miedema, Ranchor, & Kempen, 2001). It can be difficult to anticipate the rate of change of each person as an alteration in function and symptoms can depend on the stage of HF, the type of intervention(s), and the domain(s) under study (Al-Kaade & Hauptman, 2001). Making decisions about the timing between testing points is critical. For example, a medication may improve QOL in the short term, but may also increase the risk of sudden death over a longer time period. Assessments can be made at different points over time for same person or can be used to differentiate between two people at a single time point. The researcher must also decide if there should be an option for the subject to give additional input if the scale being used does not capture what is important to that person about QOL issues.

Some researchers prefer to measure QOL by coupling the assessment by the patient with an objective assessment of an outside observer. For example, Meeburg (1993) described quality of life as "a feeling of overall life satisfaction, as determined by the mentally alert individual whose life is being evaluated. Other people, preferably those from outside of that person's living situation, must agree that the individual's living conditions are not life-threatening and are adequate in meeting the individual's basic needs" (p. 37).

If patients with HF are unable to assess their QOL due to cognitive changes related to pump failure to the brain or severity of the disease process, an outside observer may provide useful information a proxy especially about the more objective, concrete and observable aspects of the illness (Addington-Hall & Kalra, 2001). Assessments of symptoms impact by patients with HF were found to be underrated when compared to families and nurses, while physician's rating were lower than all of the others (Addington-Hall & Kalra, 2001).

While the focus of most research into QOL in patients with HF has been of a quantitative nature; Bosworth et al. (2004) conducted a qualitative study of HF patients' perceptions of QOL. They conducted focus groups and used constant comparison to identify the attributes of QOL. These included symptoms, role loss, affective response, coping and social support. In addition, the patients identified concern for their family, the uncertainty of the prognosis, and changing cognitive function as important issues. Changes in their lives were not always seen as deficiencies but as opportunities for personal growth. Similarly, Zambroski (2003) used naturalistic inquiry to study women and men with living with HF. She found that the patients used language related to wind and water which she found to be a metaphor for living with HF. Categories of findings included experiencing turbulence, navigating and finding a safe harbor.

## Measuring QOL in Women with HF

There is little research available about QOL in women with cardiac disease and this data is often in comparison to men rather than with women exclusively (Janz et al., 2001). Women with HF have been found to have greater symptom impact and poorer health status than men (Bennett, Baker, & Huster, 1998; Calvert, Freemantle, & Cleland, 2005; Friedman, 2003). Bennett, Baker, and Huster (1998) found that women had more complaints of edema, sleeplessness, and memory impairment than men. Similarly, vanJaarsveld et al. (2001) found that women with HF were older and described a worse HRQOL than women with acute myocardial infarction.

Reidinger, Dracup, and Brecht (2002) compared 691 women with HF with normative groups in the Studies of Left Ventricular Dysfunction (SOLVD), and found that women with HF have significantly decreased QOL than patients with other chronic diseases such as Parkinson's disease, hypertension, and cancer. A prior portion of this research showed that increased dyspnea, life stress, and NYHA classification in women in the SOLVD study were associated with a decreased QOL (Reidinger, Dracup, & Brecht, 2000). However, increased age was associated with an increase in general life satisfaction.

## Issues of Aging and QOL

Issues of age in patients with HF can be paradoxical. Some research has shown that younger patients with HF have poorer QOL than older patients (Hou et al., 2004) related to impaired left ventricular systolic function following myocardial infarction. Whereas, older patients with HF present with hypertension and age-related changes in cardiac structures while their left ventricular function is intact (Masoudi, Havranek, & Krumholz, 2002). Patients older than 70 years were found to have a very poor prognosis (Cicoira, Davos, Florea, Shamin, Doehner, & Coats et al., 2001). Mortality rates for HF have traditionally held solid until recently since the advent of angiotensin-converting enzyme prohibitors and more aggressive treatment of hypertension and coronary disease (Masoudi, Havranek, & Krumholz, 2002).

Older patients with acute myocardial infarction (AMI) and HF were compared over a one year period, and it was found that the patients with HF were older and had worse HRQOL. While the patients with AMI were found remain stable over the year, the HRQOL of patients with HF continued to decline after diagnosis (vanJaarsveld et al., 2001). Ekman, Fagerberg, and Lundman (2002) tested elderly patients hospitalized with severe HF and found that limited functional ability and impaired QOL but also an offsetting level of sense of coherence as an internal resource. The HRQOL of elderly Chinese patients with HF was found to be most related to psychological distress, health perception, NYHA classification, and educational level (Yu, Lee, & Woo, 2004).

## QOL of Rural Dwellers

Rural Americans describe more chronic conditions and report that they are in poorer health than their urban counterparts (Ricketts, Johnson-Webb, & Randolph, 1999). Part of this issue may be limited access to health care (Schur & Franco, 1999). Employment patterns and insurance coverage complicate payment for rural health care. Lack of transportation and extended travel times may also contribute to access to health care. Access to medical specialists is often altered in rural areas and this is especially true in technology-intensive specialties such as cardiology (Schur & Franco, 1999). While the trend of closures of rural hospitals in the 1980s and 1990s has abated, rural hospitals may not offer a full range of services and thus necessitate travel to hospitals in areas with larger populations (Ricketts & Heaphy, 1999).

While access to specialized health care is often deficient in rural area, health care available in homes is similarly lacking. Borders, Aday, and Xu (2004) assessed health care accessibility, the need for assistance with ADLs, service use, social capitol, human capital, health care resources, and health status of more than 5,000 elders in a largely rural area of west Texas. While the sickest persons were older than 75 years, had less than a high school education, were retired or unemployed, and had a low household income, there were no differences in QOL found by frontier, rural, or urban residence. The authors raised the issue of whether access to health care can be associated with health status.

In contrast, Goins and Mitchell (1999) studied over 2000 adults over 60 years of age living in eastern North Carolina to discover if rurality influenced HRQOL. They assessed self-rated physical and mental health, depression, ADL's, chronic illness burden and activity levels. Significantly lower levels of QOL were found in those living in more rural areas as evidenced by more chronic illness interference, poorer self-rated mental health and higher levels of depression.

## Conclusion

Optimal health for rural dwellers remains a considerable challenge for health care providers and rural communities. Efforts to better understand the dimensions of QOL as impacted by rural dwelling as well as the aging process need further explication. Careful attention to prevent confusion about the definition and measurement of QOL must be factored into any research design. Because of the attention paid in our society to QOL issues, it can be expected that health care providers will continue to need to show evidence that interventions not only improve biological markers but QOL markers as well. Assessment of QOL can provide a powerful insight into quality of care. As health care providers work in rural communities, attention to QOL of the individual and the community at large remains a paramount concern.

### REFERENCES

Addington-Hall, J., & Kalra, L. (2001). Measuring quality of life: Who should measure quality of life? *British Medical Journal, 322,* 1417–20.

Al-Kaade, S. & Hauptman, P. (2001). Health-related quality of life measurement in heart failure: Challenges for the new millennium. *Journal of Heart Failure, 7*(2), 194–201.

Anderson, K., & Burckhardt, C. (1999). Conceptualization and measurement of quality of life as an outcome variable for health care intervention and research. *Journal of Advanced Nursing, 29*(2), 298–306.

Bennett, S., Baker, S., & Huster, G. (1998). Quality of life in women with heart failure. *Health Care for Women International, 19,* 217–229.

Bergner, M., Bobbitt, R., Carter, W., & Gilson, B. (1981). The sickness impact profile: Development and final revision of a health status measure. *Medical Care, 19,* 787–805.

Borders, T., Aday, L., & Xu, K. (2004). Factors associated with health-related quality of life among older populations in a largely rural western region. *The Journal of Rural Health, 20*(1), 67–75.

Bosworth, H., Steinhauser, K., Orr, M., Lindquist, J., Grambow, S., & Oddone, E. (2004). Congestive heart failure patients' perceptions of quality of life: The integration of physical and psychosocial factors. *Aging and Mental Health, 8*(1), 83–91.

Calvert, M., Freemantle, N., & Cleland, J. (2005). The impact of chronic heart failure in health-related quality of life data acquired at the baseline phase of the CARE-HF study. *European Journal of Heart Failure, 7*(2), 243–251.

Chin, M., & Goldman, L. (1998). Gender differences in 1-year survival and quality of life among patients admitted with congestive heart failure. *Medical Care, 36*, 1033–1046.

Chung, M., Killingworth, A., & Nolan, P. (1997). A critique of the concept of quality of life. *International Journal of Health Care Quality Assurance, 10*(2), 80–84.

Cicoira, M., Davos, C., Florea, V., Shamin, W., Doehner, W., Coats, A., et al. (2001). Chronic heart failure in the very elderly: Clinical status, survival, and prognostic factors in 188 patients more than 70 years old. *American Heart Journal, 142*, 174–180.

Corless, I., Nicholas, P., & Nokes, K. (2001) Issues in cross-cultural quality-of-life research. *Journal of Nursing Scholarship, 33*(1), 15–20.

Ekman, I., Fagerberg, B., Lundman, B. (2002). Health-related quality of life and sense of coherence among elderly patients with severe heart failure in comparison with healthy controls. *Heart & Lung, 31*, 94–101.

EuroQoL. (n.d.). How to use EQ-5D. Retrieved 5/14/2005 from http://www.euroqol.org/web/users/howtouse.php

Federal Office of Rural Health Policy & National Rural Health Association. (1998). *Rural Health. A vision for 2010.* Washington, DC: Authors.

Friedman, M. (2003). Gender differences in the health related quality of life of older adults with heart failure. *Heart & Lung, 32*, 320–327.

Gill, T., & Feinstein, A. (1994). A critical appraisal of the quality of quality-of-life measurements. *JAMA, 272*, 619–626.

Goins, R. & Mitchell, J. (1999). Health-related quality if life: Does rurality matter? *Journal of Rural Health, 15*(2), 147–156.

Guyatt, G., Feeny, D., & Patrick, D. (1993). Measuring health-related quality of life. *Annals of Internal Medicine, 118*, 622–629.

Haas, B. (1999). Clarification and integration of similar quality of life concepts. *Image: Journal of Nursing Scholarship, 31*, 215–220.

Havranek, E., Lapuerta, P., Simon, T., L'Italien, G., Block, A., & Rouleau, J. (2001). A health perceptions score predicts cardiac events in patients with heart failure: Results from the IMPRESS trial. *Journal of Cardiac Failure, 7*(2), 153–157.

Hou, N., Chui, M., Eckert, G., Oldridge, N., Murray, M., & Bennett, S. (2004). Relationship of age and sex to health-related quality of life in patients with heart failure. *American Journal of Critical Care, 13*, 153–161.

Janz, N., Janevic, M., Dodge, J., Fingerlin, T., Schork, A., Mosca, L., et al. (2001). Factors influencing quality of life in older women with heart disease. *Medical Care, 39*(6), 588–598.

Kaplan, R. (1988). Health-related quality of life in cardiovascular disease. *Journal of Consulting and Clinical Psychology, 56*(3), 2.

Karnofsky, D. & Burchenal, J. (1949). The clinical evaluation of chemotherapeutic agents in cancer. In C. Macleod (Ed.), *Evaluation of chemotherapeutic agents* (p. 196). New York: Columbia University.

Katz, S., Ford, A., Moskowitz, R., Jackson, B., & Jaffe, M. (1963). Studies of illness in the aged. *JAMA, 185*, 914–919.

Kinney, M., Burfitt, S., Stullenburger, E., Rees, B., & DeBolt, M. (1996). Quality of life in cardiac patient research: A meta-analysis. *Nursing Research, 45*(3), 173–180.

Konstram, M., Dracup, K., Baker, D., Bottordoff, M., Brooks, N., Dacey, R., et al. (1995). *Heart failure: Evaluation and care of patients with left-ventricular dysfunction. Clinical practice guidelines No. 11* (AHCPR Publication No. 94–0612. Rockville, MD: U.S. Department of Health and Human Services.

Lawton, M., & Brody, E. (1969). Assessment of older people: Self-maintaining and instrumental activities of daily living. *Gerontologist, 9*, 179–186.

Mapi Research Trust. (2004). Patient-reported outcome and quality of life database. Retrieved May 16, 2005 from: http://proqolid.org/ind_home2004.html

Maramaldi, P., Berkman, B., &, Barusch. A. (2005). Assessment and the ubiquity of culture: Threats to validity in measures of health-related quality of life. *Health and Social Work, 30*(1), 27–39.

Masoudi, F., Havranek, E., & Krumholz, H. (2002). The burden of chronic congestive heart failure in older persons: Magnitude and implications for policy and research. *Heart Failure Review, 7*(1), 9–16.

Meeburg, G. (1993). Quality of life: A concept analysis. *Journal of Advanced Nursing, 18*, 32–38.

Moons, P. (2004). Why call it health-related quality of life when you mean perceived health status? *European Journal of Cardiovascular Nursing, 3*(4), 275–277.

Online Guide to QOL Instruments (OGLA). Retrieved May 25, 2005 from http://www.ogla-qol.com

President's Commission of National Goals: Goals for America. (1960). Columbia University: The American Assembly, NY.

Prutkin, J. & Feinstein, A. (2002). Quality-of-life measurements: Origin and pathogenesis. *Yale Journal of Biology and Medicine, 75*, 79–93.

Rector, T., & Cohn, J. (1992). Assessment of patient outcome with the Minnesota living with heart failure questionnaire: Reliability and validity during a randomized, double-blind, placebo-controlled trial of pimobendan. *American Heart Journal, 124*, 1017–1025.

Rector, T., Tschumperlin, L., Kubo, S., Bank, A., Francis, G., McDonald, K., et al. (1995). Use of the living with heart failure questionnaire to ascertain patient's perspectives on improvement in quality of life versus risk of drug-induced death. *Journal of Cardiac Failure, 1*(3), 201–206.

Reidinger, M., Dracup, K., & Brecht, M. (2000). Predictors of quality of life in women with heart failure. *Journal of Heart and Lung Transplant, 19*, 598–608.

Reidinger, M., Dracup, K., & Brecht, M. (2002). Quality of life in women with heart failure, normative groups, and patients with other conditions. *American Journal of Critical Care, 11*(3), 211–220.

Ricketts, T., & Heaphy, S. (1999). Access to health care. In T. Ricketts (Ed.), *Rural health in the United States* (pp. 101–112). New York: Oxford University.

Ricketts, T., Johnson-Webb, K., & Randolph, R. (1999). Populations and places in rural America. In T. Ricketts (Ed.), *Rural health in the United States* (pp. 7–24). New York: Oxford University.

Schur, C., & Franco, S. (1999). Access to health care. In T. Ricketts (Ed.), *Rural health in the United States* (pp. 25–37). New York: Oxford University.

Staniszewska, S., Ahmed, L., & Jenkinson, C. (1999). The conceptual validity and appropriateness of using health-related quality of life measures with minority groups. *Ethnicity & Health, 4*(1/2), 51–64.

Stull, D., Clough, L., & Van Dussen, D. (2001). Self-report quality of life as a predictor of hospitalization for patients with LV dysfunction: A life course approach. *Research in Nursing and Health, 24*, 460–469.

vanJaarsveld, C., Sanderman, R., Miedema, I., Ranchor, A., & Kempen, G. (2001). Changes in health-related quality of life in older patients with acute myocardial infarction of congestive heart failure: A prospective study. *Journal of the American Geriatric Society, 49*, 1052–1058.

Ware, J., & Sherbourne, C. (1992). The MOS short-form health survey (SF36). 1. Conceptual framework and item selection. *Medical Care, 30*, 473–483.

Westlake, C., Dracup, K., Creaser, J., Livingston, N., Heywood, T., Huiskes, B., et al. (2002). Correlates of health-related quality of life in patients with heart failure. *Heart & Lung, 31*(2), 85–93.

World Health Organization. (1948). Preamble to the Constitution of the World Health Organization. Geneva: Author.

Yu, D., Lee, D., & Woo, J. (2004). Health-related quality of life in elderly Chinese patients with heart failure. *Research in Nursing and Health, 27*, 332–344.

Zambroski, C. (2003). Qualitative analysis of living with heart failure. *Heart & Lung, 32*, 32–40.

*Chapter 9*

# *Notification of Eligibility for Hospice Services for Terminally Ill Pulmonary Disease, End-Stage Renal Disease, and Amyotrophic Lateral Sclerosis Inpatients at a University Hospital*

MELANIE KALMAN AND ROBERTA ROLLAND

**Abstract:** Hospice is an important service that is beneficial to terminally ill patients. This descriptive study using retrospective chart review included examination of 124 charts of end stage pulmonary disease (ESPD), end stage renal disease (ESRD), and (ALS) patients and found that patients are frequently not notified or are infrequently notified about eligibility for hospice services. If patients and their families are not notified or notified late in the patient's disease process than they can not avail themselves of all hospice services. Thus, it is important to identify whether or not patients and their families are appropriately notified about hospice services in a timely manner. While the physician is the gate keeper for hospice admission, the nurse also has a pivotal role in recognizing when hospice services would be useful.

## Introduction

Hospice is recognized as a way to provide comprehensive services for dying patients and their families. However, patients are often not admitted to hospice early enough to use the services effectively. Whether this is because patients who are eligible are not being notified about hospice or are not notified until it is too late to benefit from hospice services have not been well documented in the literature. At one hospice in central New York two trends have been identified. The first is towards an increase in the number of patients referred to hospice who die before they can be admitted and the second is an increase in the number of patients who die within one week of admission to hospice (Borstelmann 1996; Stewart, personal communication, 2002). It is hypothesized in this study that patients are admitted late in the course of their terminal disease because they are not notified about the availability of hospice services until late in their disease. Issues surrounding cancer patients and hospice have been previously studied. However, terminal illnesses go beyond the spectrum of cancer. Although there are clear, well written admission criteria for terminally ill pulmonary disease (ESPD), end-stage renal disease (ESRD), and amyotrophic lateral sclerosis (ALS) patients, the hospice admission rates for these patients have not been examined. The purpose of this study is to document whether hospitalized patients terminally ill with pulmonary disease, end-stage renal disease, and amyotrophic lateral sclerosis who are eligible for hospice services have documented hospice notification in their charts.

## Literature Review

Kubler-Ross wrote that "death is still a fearful, frightening happening and the fear of death is a universal fear" (Kubler-Ross, 1969, p. 5). Although death itself is universal, the cause of death changed throughout the 1900s. Until the mid twentieth century an infectious disease was commonly the cause of death. With the advent of antibiotics after World War II, death from infectious disease decreased. Today death is more commonly caused by complications from chronic illnesses. Concurrent with change in etiology there was an upsurge in technological advances in healthcare. Because of technological advances in the delivery of health care medicine's focus shifted from comfort to cure. This shift created problems when cure was not possible. If there were no pills or technology to cure, the healthcare system was at a loss as to it's role. The concept of hospice was developed in response to problems seen with end-of-life care. Although the concept of hospice dates back to the early 1900s, it was more fully developed in the 1960s by Dr. Cicely Saunders at St. Christopher's Hospice in London (Lichter, 1984). The hospice movement took root in the United States (U.S.) with the first U.S. hospice established in 1974 in Connecticut (Friedrich, 1999). The hospice philosophy includes the beliefs that dying is a normal process and that through appropriate care, patients and their families may be free to attain a degree of preparation for death that is satisfactory to them (National Hospice and Palliative Care Organization [NHPCO], 1998).

In the U.S., due to reimbursement issues hospice is limited to the last six months of life (Ferrell & Coyle, 2001). Because of this limitation on service, U.S. patients are not receiving the full possible benefit of hospice. In addition, if referral is not made in a timely manner benefit from hospice services can be extremely curtailed or even negated. Early on, Lichter (1984) identified the need for change regarding reimbursement of Medicare and Medicaid to decrease barriers to hospice. Other countries with socialized health coverage, including Canada and the United Kingdom, do not have such time barriers. Therefore transition to hospice care services is less difficult in these countries (Lichter, 1984).

Naik and DeHaven (2001) state that while third party payers allow for six months of hospice benefits, the average hospice patient receives one month of services. Stillman and Syrjala (1999) found that the mean length of stay in one hospice was 55 days, with a median of 23 days. A hospice in central New York the average and median length of stay decreased by 25–30% in 1994 to 1995 (Borstelmann 1996). Furthermore, in 1999 12% of patients referred to hospice died before they could be admitted. This figure rose to 13.5% in 2000. In 1998 five percent of hospice referrals died within two days and six percent died within one week of admission (Stewart, personal communication, 2002). In one study, Emanuel, von Gunten, and Ferris (2000) found that the median stay for hospice dropped from 36 in 1995 to fewer than 20 days in 1998. "For several years the declining average length of stay in hospice and the growth in the proportion of very-short stay patients has been one of the biggest challenges for hospice providers. At the local level, providers seek to educate referral sources about the poor outcomes of late referrals, while on the national level the NHPCO is seeking to find alternative eligibility criteria than Medicare's six-month-or-less requirement" (Davie, 1999, p. 5).

Many authors have identified physicians as the primary gatekeepers of hospice but found that they delay in admitting patients to hospice (Hyman & Bulkin, 1990; Lamont & Christakis, 2001). Three reasons that physicians may delay suggesting hospice to patients are their own difficulties with death, a perception that they will lose control over medical decisions for their patients, and the difficulty in predicting when a patient has reached the final six months of their illness. First, it may be as difficult for health care professionals to face death as it is for laypersons. It is certainly difficult to tell a patient and their family that they have a terminal disease. It is even more difficult to say s/he has six months or less to live. This may lead to what Travis (2004) called treatment futility. This is defined as offering treatment when one believes it will not help because one believes that this is what the family wishes.

The second reason, the fear of loss of control over medical decisions, was cited by Massarotto, Carter, Macleod, and Donaldson (2000). They reported that over one-third of physicians in their study were wary of hospice since they felt that they would lose the right to make medical decisions for their patients. In addition physicians expressed feelings that they were not ready to discontinue all curative treatments.

The third reason physicians delay in suggesting hospice is the difficulty in predicting death. Lamont and Christakis (2001) found that physician's predictions of survival in their terminally ill patients were often inaccurate (80%) and usually optimistic (63%). Optimistic estimates may lead to treatment futility rather than more appropriate supportive care. Predicting when a patient has reached the final six months of their illness is more challenging for terminal patients with non-cancer diagnoses, since cancer is somewhat more predictable than some other diseases (O'Brien, 2002). Christakis and Escarce (1996) reported in 1990 that less than 20% of referrals to hospice in five major states carried a non-cancer diagnosis. Miller, Weitzen, and Kinzbrunner (2003) found that the probability of a short hospice stay (7 days or less) was greater for patients with non-cancer diagnoses.

A fourth reason that physicians may not refer patients to hospice is because many medical schools do not discuss this important concept. The American Medical Association found that only four of 126 U.S. medical schools required a separate course on caring for the dying. The lack of education in medical schools led to the development of Education for Physicians in End-of-Life Care (EPEC), a project intended to equip physicians with a core base of knowledge need for end-of-life care (Emanuel et al., 2000).

While the physician is the health care team member to order hospice referrals, the nurse also has a considerable role when patients are making the decision for hospice care. One reason for the considerable role is because nurses spend more time with terminal patients than any other member of the health care team. The nurse serves as the primary liaison between the health care team and the patient and family, advocates for the patient, coordinates the complex care, including symptom management, addresses the psychosocial and spiritual aspects of care, and serves as a resource and educator by providing information about medications, equipment, and procedures (Malone, 2003; O'Brien, 2002; Puntillo, 2001). The American Association of Colleges joined forces with the City of Hope National Medical Center to address the knowledge deficits of nurses related to end-of-life care (Sherman, Matzo, Panke, Grant, & Rhome, 2003). Subsequently, the End-of-Life Nursing Education Consortium (ELNEC) was developed in 2000 with funding from the Robert Wood Johnson Foundation. It provides resources for schools of nursing and nursing agencies/organizations.

Educational programs for the healthcare professional are a step in the right direction addressing end-of-life care. However barriers remain concerning late referrals to hospice services, especially for terminally ill patients that do not have cancer. There are clear criteria, written as guidelines, for hospice admission for specified non-cancer diseases. End stage pulmonary Disease (ESPD), End Stage Renal Disease (ESRD), and Amyotrophic Lateral Sclerosis (ALS) are among the non-cancer disease guidelines identified by NHPCO (1998) and were the diagnoses chosen for this study. Before patients can choose hospice services one needs to ascertain if they were notified about their eligibility for hospice. This descriptive study examined the hospice notification rates for ESPD, ESRD, and ALS.

## Methods

This descriptive retrospective chart review design study was conducted in order to answer the following research question. When terminally ill hospitalized ESPD, ESRD, and ALS patients meet the criteria for hospice admission, are they notified about hospice by healthcare professionals?

### Sample

After careful consideration and discussions with the local hospice agency and the local palliative care service, it was decided that terminally ill ESPD, ESRD, and ALS hospitalized patients should comprise the sample for this study. A total of 124 charts were reviewed of patients who were admitted to a university health science center over a six month period and who had a coded diagnosis of one of the following diagnosis: pulmonary disease and who were on a ventilator, ESRD or ALS. Of the 124 charts that were reviewed 71 (57.3%) ESPD patients, 49 (39.5%) ESRD patients and 4 (3.2%) were ALS patients. Fifty-seven (46%) were female and 67 (54%) were male.

## Data Collection

Approval to conduct this exploratory, descriptive design using retrospective chart review was obtained from the Institutional Review Board. Clinical Data Services generated a list of all inpatients over the age of 18 years admitted to a university medical center between January 1, 2002 and June 30, 2002 with selected diagnoses. The principal investigator (PI), reviewed the list for multiple admissions and deleted the earlier admissions from the list. This ensured that the same patient was not counted twice. A total of 124 charts of ESPD, ESRD, and ALS hospitalized patients who may have been eligible for hospice were reviewed. All charts of ESPD patients requiring ventilator support and ALS patients were reviewed. Randomly chosen ESRD patients (20%) were reviewed. The PI chose a number from a table of random numbers and matched it to the last digits of a patient's record. This determined the first ESRD patient's chart to review. After that every fifth ESRD patient chart on the list was selected to be reviewed. Approximately two to three ventilated pulmonary disease patients, 50 ESRD patients, and two ALS are admitted monthly to the university hospital. Reviewing all of the charts of the ventilated pulmonary disease patient sample, 20% of the ESRD patients, and all of the charts of the ALS patients equalized the number of charts examined in each category. Unique patient identifiers, such as name and social security numbers, were not collected nor were patients or their families contacted.

The research team consisted of the authors plus four nursing students enrolled at a College of Nursing Masters' program. The PI reviewed the first charts to determine feasibility of the tool. All reviewers were trained by the PI and inter-rater reliability was reached when the PI reviewed charts with each reviewer and attained similar results.

Notification of Eligibility for Hospice Services

## Instruments

Since the study examined local eligibility for hospice admission the tools were based on the local hospice admission criteria. The local hospice admission policy is based on criteria from the National Hospice and Palliative Care Organization (NHPCO). The admission criteria were rewritten as a tool (see Figure 1). The tool was reviewed by an expert for content validity. Demographic data including gender, age, diagnosis, ethnicity, insurance, and religion were also obtained.

**Figure 1**
*Admissions Criteria for Hospice of Central NY:
Amyotrophic Lateral Sclerosis*

---

Progression of ALS differs markedly from patient to patient. The rate of progression in a given patient is very important in estimating prognosis. Two other critical factors for admission eligibility are respiratory function and ability to swallow.

1. Rapid progression of disease as evidenced by
significant changes in performance status (bed bound) yes ____ no ____
significant changes in speech yes ____ no ____
significant changes in ability to swallow yes ____ no ____
2. Respiratory function — patient has compromised respiratory function and does not want mechanical ventilation. yes ____ no ____
requires supplemental $O^2$ yes ____ no ____
significant decrease in $FEV_1$ yes ____ no ____
shortness of breath with exertion yes ____ no ____
unable to raise secretions and/or has a cough yes ____ no ____
3. Ability to swallow
oral intake insufficient to sustain life yes ____ no ____
patient doesn't want artificial feeding yes ____ no ____
progressive weight loss yes ____ no ____
Other factors which may shorten progression
recurrent aspiration pneumonia yes ____ no ____
decubitis ulcer(s), stage 3–4 yes ____ no ____
urinary tract/ kidney infection yes ____ no ____
sepsis yes ____ no ____
fever recurrent after antibiotics yes ____ no ____
Informed of hospice yes ____ no ____
By whom (title) _____
Date of notification _____

*(Form based on admission criteria of Hospice of Central NY)*

## Data Analysis

Data were analyzed using non-parametric, descriptive statistics in an aggregate format so that patients were not identifiable. Individual data was known only to the research team. The computer program, SPSS version 12, was used.

## Results

Results showed that of the 124 in-patient hospital charts reviewed, nine patients were eligible for hospice (7.3%). Of the nine eligible patients, five (55%) were informed of hospice services. Of the five informed, one (20%) died before discharge from the hospital. Of the four patients that were eligible and not informed, two (50%) died before hospital discharge (see Figure 2).

**Figure 2**
*Patients Eligible for Hospice and Informed*
*(n=9)*

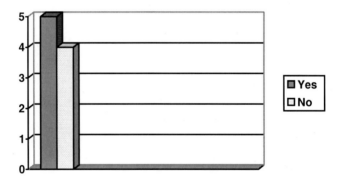

## Discussion

In this study nine patients were found to be eligible for hospice admission and only five were informed of their eligibility. The findings of this study are supported by the literature. When notification does occur, often there is not enough time to receive the full benefit of hospice services. Hospice services, such as symptom management and bereavement counseling, are processes that require time. Nurses in hospitals as well as community settings are in a pivotal position to recognize when hospice services would be useful. Furthermore, many nurses, in a variety of practice settings, are intimately involved with end of life care but may be unaware that patients and their families are frequently not told about this important service. Because patients and families often seek information from nurses, nursing is in a key position to assume a proactive role in end of life care by determining whether terminally ill patients are aware of hospice services that are available. When patients or families express an interest in hospice, nurses can advocate and facilitate discussions with their primary care providers.

Further research is needed to ascertain why healthcare professionals delay informing patients and their families about hospice and the services they offer. If the problem is reimbursement issues then extending reimbursement beyond six months for hospice services or reimbursing for palliative care may result in earlier admissions. Other nations employ the hospice concept without the six month clause to qualify for eligibility. Perhaps changes are needed at the federal level. If the problem is issues surrounding death in American culture then programs such as EPEC or ELNEC will help teach health care professionals how to initiate conversations with patients and families about end of life issues.

The limitations to this study include the nature of chart documentation. It is believed that more than nine of the 124 inpatients were eligible for hospice service since some of the reviewers also worked in the hospital where the charts were reviewed. However, if a chart did not have the needed documentation, those patients were not counted as eligible for hospice services. A concurrent review would have given a more accurate picture of who was eligible but would have been more costly.

## Conclusion

Hospice provides unique services for terminally ill patients. Unless patients are notified they can not make the decision whether or not to use these services and will lose out on valuable services. The nurse is in a unique position to advocate for notifying patients of their eligibility. As one author aptly states, "The only failure in therapy for terminally ill patients is the failure to refer hospice as the next step in health care" (Gloth, 1998, p. 5).

## NOTE

This study was funded with an internal grant from the Upstate Medical University College of Nursing.

## REFERENCES

Borstelmann, L. (1996). Hospice programs struggle with declining lengths of stays. *The DOH Advisor*. Syracuse, NY: State Department of Health.

Christakis, N. A., & Escarce, J. J. (1996). Survival of Medicare patients after enrollment in hospice programs. *The New England Journal of Medicine, 335(3)*, 172–8.

Davie, K. (1999, Fall). Preserving hospice's core values in an environment of change. *The Hospice Professional*. Alexandria, VA: National Council of Hospice Professionals.

Emanuel, L., von Gunten, C., & Ferris, F. (2000). Gaps in end-of-life care. *Archives of Family Medicine, 9*(10), 1176–80.

Ferrell, B. R., & Coyle, N. (2001). *Textbook of palliative care nursing*. New York: Oxford University.

Friedrich, M. J., (1999). Hospice care in the United States: A conversation with Florence S. Wald. *JAMA, 281*, 1683–5.

Gloth, M. (1998). Forward. In National Hospice and Palliative Care Organization, *Hospice care: A physician's guide*. Alexandra, VA: National Council of Hospice Professionals.

Hyman, B., H., & Bulkin, W. (1990). Physician reported incentives and disincentives for referring patients to hospice. *The Hospice Journal, 6*(4), 39–64.

Kubler-Ross E. (1969). *On Death and Dying*. New York, NY: Macmillan.

Lamont, E. B, and Christakis, N. A. (2001). Prognostic disclosure to patients with cancer near the end of life. *Annals of Internal Medicine, 134*(12), 1096–1105.

Lichter, I. (1984). Specialist palliative-care services. In D. Doyle, *Palliative care: The management of far-advanced illness*. Philadelphia: The Charles.

Malone, B. (2003). Getting it right: Beverly Malone on nurse prescribing and end-of life issues. *Nursing Standard, 17*(42), 26.

Massarotto, P., Carter, H., Macleod, R., & Donaldson, N. (2000). Hospital referrals to a hospice: Timing of referrals, referrers', expectations, and the nature of referral information. *Journal of Palliative Care, 16*(3), 22–9.

Miller, S. C., Weitzen, S., & Kinzbrunner, B. (2003). Factors associated with higher prevalence of short hospice stays. *Journal of Palliative Medicine, 6*(5), 725–36.

Naik, A., & DeHaven, M. J. (2001). Short stays in Hospice: A review and update. *Caring, 20*(2), 10–3.

National Hospice and Palliative Care Organization (1998). *Hospice care: A physician's guide.* Alexandria, VA: National Council of Hospice Professionals.

O'Brien, N. (2002). *Nursing care at the end of life.* Sacramento: CME Resource.

Puntillo, K. (2001). Symptom management at end of life: The importance of nursing. *American Nurse, 33*(3), 19.

Sherman, D. W., Matzo, M. L., Panke, J., Grant, M., & Rhome, A. (2003). End-of-life nursing education consortium curriculum: An introduction to palliative care. *Nurse Educator, 28*(3), 111–20.

Stillman, M. & Syrjarla, K. (1999). Differences in physician access patterns to hospice care. *Journal of Pain and Symptom Management, 17*(3), 157–63.

Travis S. (2004, March). *Reframing end-of-life care.* Paper presented at the annual meeting of National Association of Clinical Nurse Specialists, San Antonio, TX.

*Chapter 10*

# Sexual Behavior Patterns of Rural Men who Have Sex with Men: Description and Implications for Intervention

ANTHONY R. D'AUGELLI, DEBORAH BRAY PRESTON, RICHARD E. CAIN, AND FREDERICK W. SCHULZE

**Abstract:** Few studies investigate sexual behavior patterns of men who have sex with men (MSM) living in rural areas. Little is known about the nature of these MSM's relationships, their sexual partners, or their sexual behavior, especially behavior that would increase their risk for HIV infection. This exploratory study describes the relationships of 99 rural MSM, their sexual partners, and their sexual experiences. Partner characteristics, locations for meeting partners, prevalence of risky behavior, reasons for engaging in risky sexual behavior, and efforts to decrease risk, were assessed. Results indicated that over half had multiple sexual partners in the last six months, and over one-third had anonymous partners. Nearly half reported unprotected receptive anal intercourse with their primary partners, 13% with casual partners, and 25% with anonymous partners. About one-quarter were categorized as being at high risk for HIV infection. Implications for future preventive interventions designed for rural MSM are discussed.

Little research has been conducted on men who have sex with men (MSM) who reside in rural areas (Preston, D'Augelli, Cain, & Schulze, 2002). The major early studies of sexual orientation (e.g., Bell, Weinberg, & Hammersmith, 1981) as well as much of the more contemporary research that describes same-sex sexual attractions, behavior, and identity have been conducted in urban areas in which there are considerably higher populations of lesbian, gay, and bisexual adults as compared to suburban or rural areas (Berry, 2000; Laumann, Gagnon, Michael, & Michaels, 1994). Access to research participants is easier in non-rural areas, and the prevalence of HIV in metropolitan areas has directed the focus of past research. Although there is some evidence that supports the phenomenon of lesbian, gay, and bisexual people who grew up in rural or suburban areas migrating to cities in which they can live more openly (D'Augelli & Hart, 1987; D'Augelli, Preston, Kassab, & Cain, 2002), the strong stigma attached to same-sex sexual orientation in rural areas makes estimates of the numbers of MSM living in non-metropolitan parts of the country very difficult. The characteristics and personal issues associated with this population have not been described, nor has their risk for HIV infection been delineated (Cohn, 1997).

The CDC's HIV Prevention Strategy for 2001 to 2005 has as its primary goal decreasing the number of people at high risk for HIV infection by at least 50% through helping communities mobilize preventive education and ancillary services (CDC, *HIV Prevention Strategic Plan*, 2001). This goal is most important in rural areas of America; where HIV/AIDS issues are critical in the face of increasing numbers of persons with HIV/AIDS, and the restricted care available (Schur et al., 2002). MSM who live in rural areas are a diverse and hidden population. Some identify as gay or bisexual, but some do not, despite engaging in same-sex sexual experiences. Some are in same-sex partnerships, some of which do not involve cohabitation; some are single; and, some are heterosexually partnered or married. The expression of sexual orientation for these men, however, can be very different from that of their urban counterparts. The most important differences can be traced to the broad contextual differences between urban and rural life. For rural MSM, social isolation and a lack of networking opportunities with other MSM are common (Lindhorst, 1997; Mancoske, 1997; Preston et al., 2002; Smith, 1997). Although stigma, rejection, and social isolation are also present among MSM in urban areas, the anonymity associated with higher population density in cities means that gay and bisexual men are more likely to be "connected" to a gay community. Moreover, urban men may have much less fear about the disclosure of their sexual orientation to families and friends. Not only is it much less likely that urban men's families will see them in a gay-identified venue or with gay friends (anonymity and the multiple venues available contribute to this safety), but it is also more likely that they have potential access to more support from others if their sexual orientation does become known and their families respond negatively. In many cities, there are specific neighborhoods containing high concentrations of lesbians, gay men, and bisexual people, with a social and cultural infrastructure to serve them (Garnets & D'Augelli, 1994).

This is not the case in rural settings where the opportunity structure for the development of one's sexual orientation has distinct limitations (D'Augelli & Hart, 1987; D'Augelli, Hart, & Collins, 1987; D'Augelli et al., 2002). Places for social and sexual contact are far fewer; the ability to develop close same-sex friendships or romantic relationships in an open way is compromised; and the chance for the development of a gay community consisting of formal and informal social networks is undercut by powerful forces reinforcing invisibility. Another important factor in the lives of rural MSM is the possibility of rejection from family and friends. Others' knowledge of one's sexual orientation can occur thanks to the "small town grapevine," which makes it difficult to maintain privacy in many important life domains (Martinez-Brawley & Blundall, 1989). Even persons closely associated with rural MSM, such as family members and personal friends, may be at risk for social rejection if men's sexual orientation becomes known (Mayne & O'Leary, 1993). For example, Anderson and Lane-Shaw (1994) found that stigma that included fear of social disapproval, a blemish on family identity, or loss of prestige in the community, were reasons given by family members for not disclosing the sexual orientation of a relative. Unfortunately, rejection of rural MSM by some family members, if not their entire families, is not uncommon (Preston et al., 2004; Sowell & Christensen, 1996; Weitz, 1991). Many MSM living in rural areas cannot afford to risk rejection and ostracism from family, friends, and others in their communities, and hide their sexual orientation as a means of survival. Because of this, many rural MSM internalize feelings of social rejection, and internalized homophobia can develop (Smith, 1997). This form of cultural and social oppression has been shown to be related to self-esteem and mental health problems (Herek, Cogan, Gillis, & Glunt, 1998; Kus & Smith, 1995; Shidlo, 1994).

The purpose of this study was to describe the sexual behavior patterns of a sample of rural MSM. Particular focus was placed on relationship patterns, the number and types of sexual partners men had, and the sexual activities they engaged in with different kinds of sexual partners. Behaviors that increase risk of HIV infection were surveyed, and ways men attempted to avoid HIV infection were queried. Communication patterns with sexual partners about HIV risk reduction behaviors were included, as was men's experiences with

HIV testing. Although there is no presumption that ours is a representative sample of rural MSM, this exploratory analysis of their sexual behavior patterns was expected to shed light on the potential impact of the rural context on their sexual behavior.

## Method

### Participants

Participants were 99 MSM living in rural Pennsylvania who ranged in age from 18 to 69 years ($M = 37.8$, $SD = 11.3$). Most (95%) were Caucasian and were employed full time (80%).

### Sampling

Because we were unable to obtain a random sample or a representative sample, we accessed potential participants through other men who were trusted friends, or through several informal social networks, which are common ways for rural gay and bisexual men to meet in rural areas (D'Augelli & Hart, 1987).

Respondents were recruited from those attending social activities for gay and bisexual men, local gay bars, and gay pride events. These events were not publicly advertised, but were announced through newsletters, private electronic mail lists, and word-of-mouth.

### Data Collection

Rural residence was verified by having the men identify the county in which they resided and their zip code. Of the 66 counties in Pennsylvania, approximately 50 have been designated as non-metropolitan based on population density and distance from a metropolitan area. Only men residing in one of these 50 counties and whose zip code was classified as rural were recruited (Center for Rural Pennsylvania, 2001).

At the social gatherings, men were asked by members of the research team to fill out a questionnaire, seal it in an envelope, and place it in a sealed box. Participants were provided with an informed consent form which they read prior to completing the questionnaire. No names or identifying information were included in their responses, and the questionnaires were not opened until the data collection from all sites was complete, thus assuring confidentiality. Respondents were provided a small honorarium for participating. On the average, the instrument required 20 minutes to complete.

## *Measures*

### *Personal Characteristics*

Respondents were asked their age, racial/ethnic background, level of education, income, and other background characteristics. They were asked to describe their sexual orientation based on a seven-point Kinsey-type scale of sexual attraction, with "6" indicating completely same-sex oriented, and "0" indicating completely heterosexual.

### *Relationship Status*

First, respondents were asked if they were in a long term relationship with another person that has lasted at least six months. They were asked the gender of this partner, the nature of the relationship (a committed couple, dating, or likely to become a committed couple), the duration of the relationship, whether or not the men cohabited. Men who stated that they were not in a relationship during the last six months were defined as single for the purposes of the study.

### *Methods for Meeting Sexual Partners*

Whether or not the respondent had met other men for sexual experiences in the following ways was asked: through personal ads or dating services, at a health club or gym, at a public venue (park, rest stop, restroom), over the Internet such as through a chat room, in a gay public entertainment setting (bar, night club, dance club), at private parties, through friends, or at work.

## Sexual Partners

Following questions concerning their relationship status, men in relationships were asked about their and their partner's sexual involvement with others. They were asked if they or their partners had other sexual partners during the course of their relationship ("Yes," "No," or "Don't Know").

Questions were later asked about the type and number of sexual partners the men had in the last six months. Sexual partners were defined as other people with whose sex organs the participant had direct contact. The gender of the partners was sought. Three types of partners were defined: "primary partners," including a steady partner, "casual partners," regular sexual partners who were known to the respondent, but who were not steady partners, and "unknown partners," anonymous partners that the men "did not know at all." For each of the three partner types, the men provided the number of partners, and then the number who were HIV-infected (HIV positive), uninfected with HIV (HIV negative), and whose HIV status was unknown. The lifetime number of the men's sexual partners who were HIV positive was also asked.

## Sexual Risk Behavior

Questions about specific sexual behavior also focused on the last six months. Four types of sexual behavior were of interest: receptive anal sex without a condom, receptive anal sex with a condom, insertive anal sex without a condom, and insertive anal sex with a condom. For each activity, men estimated the frequency of behavior with primary partners, causal partners, and unknown partners. Four options were used to describe the frequency of each behavior with different types of partners: "no such partners," "never do this," "do this sometimes," or "do this every time."

The riskiness of sexual behavior patterns was measured by the Coping and Change Sexual Behavior Questionnaire (CCSBQ; Ostrow, DiFranceisco, & Wagstaff, 1998). The CCSBQ assesses levels of sexual risk related to partner type (primary or steady; partners who are well-known but not steady; casual acquaintances who are not anonymous; and anonymous partners), number of partners, condom use (every time, sometimes, never), and frequency of receptive anal sex.

The instrument consists of 18 items; 6 are composed of sub-parts designed to gather information about specific sexual behaviors of MSM: rimming; receptive and insertive anal sex; receptive and insertive fellatio; and mutual masturbation. The responses to items on frequency of receptive anal sex, partner type, and use of condoms are combined into a four-level sexual risk variable (no risk, low risk, modified high risk, and high risk). A composite sexual risk variable was constructed following Ostrow et al.'s (1998) recommendations. Responses to items on frequency of receptive anal sex, partner type, and use of condoms were combined into a four-level sexual risk variable. The four categories were:

1. no risk: men who had not reported sex with another person in the last six months, or who were monogamous and not having receptive anal sex with partners.
2. low risk: men in monogamous relationships who were having receptive anal sex and who always used condoms, or men who had multiple partners but did not have receptive anal sex.
3. modified high risk: men in monogamous relationships having receptive anal sex who did not always use condoms, or men with multiple partners, who were having receptive anal sex and always used condoms
4. high risk: men who were having receptive anal sex with multiple partners who did not always use condoms. The reliability and validity of the CCSBQ have been established. (Ostrow et al.)

Because of its importance to HIV risk, an open-ended question about lifetime sexual experience with HIV positive partners was included. The question was, "In your lifetime, with how many partners who you knew to be HIV positive at the time you had sex, did you have unprotected receptive anal intercourse?"

## Personal and Interpersonal Strategies Used to Minimize Risk of HIV Infection

Men were asked how often ("always," "sometimes," or "never") they had done each of the following to reduce their risk for HIV infection: (a) was no longer the receptive partner in anal sex, (b) was only the insertive partner in anal sex, (c) avoided contact with other men's semen, (d) avoided using alcohol or drugs before sex, (e) asked potential partners about their HIV status, (f) asked potential partners about their sexual histories (number of past partners, etc.), and (g) discussed condom use prior to engaging in sex. The reliability coefficient for scores on this scale were .65.

Then they were asked how often they actually did the following before having sexual experiences with another man in the past six months: (a) asked the partner about his feelings about condom use, (b) asked the partner about the partner's number of other sexual partners, (c) told the partner about his own past number of partners, (d) told partners that he would not have anal sex without a condom, (e) discussed the need for both men to be tested for HIV before having sex, (f) talked with new partners about delaying sex until they knew each other better, (g) asked a new partner about his history of sexually transmitted infections, and (h) asked new partners about their use of injectable drugs such a heroin, speed, or cocaine.

Being tested for HIV is another strategy men use to for self-protection as well as protecting partners. Men were asked if they had ever been tested, how often they had been tested, the results of their last test, and their future plans for testing. They were asked their reasons for not having been tested if they had never been tested. Reply options related to lack of testing were: "I'm at low risk of HIV infection," "I'm scared to learn the results," "I'm scared of needles," "I don't care," and, "I don't know." Several other questions were asked using a Likert-type scale, with responses ranging from "strongly agree" to "strongly disagree." The reasons for not getting tested included: (a) fear of being seen by others, who would then know that he was gay or bisexual, (b) having been tested in the past, (c) not being concerned about HIV infection because of the new treatments available, and (d) having "faith in God that I'll be OK."

## Intoxication During Sexual Activity

For the three types of partners (primary, casual, and unknown), men were asked about their use of three types of intoxicants during sexual experiences they had within the last six months. They were asked how often they used alcohol (three or more alcoholic drinks), drugs (marijuana, cocaine, MDA, LSD, uppers, downers, K, and Ecstasy), or amyl or butyl nitrate ("poppers") when they had sex.

They were then asked if drug use other than alcohol had caused them to engage in sexual activity they later regretted. This was answered with "never," "occasionally," or "often." Those who had regrets were asked to describe their experiences.

## Assessment of Personal Risk of HIV Infection

Respondents were asked, "When you compare yourself to the average gay or bisexual man, what would you say are your chances of getting AIDS?" There were four response choices, which ranged from "much lower" through "much higher." A related question was also asked: "On a scale of 1 to 5, with 1 being not at all risky and 5 meaning extremely risky, how risky do you think your current sexual behaviors are for contracting HIV?"

## Barriers to Avoiding Unprotected Receptive Anal Intercourse

Men who have ever had receptive anal intercourse without a condom were asked to consider seven reasons this occurred: (a) "My partner would be offended," (b) "It would spoil the mood," (c) "It would reduce the pleasure," (d) "It was too much trouble," (e) "I felt embarrassed talking about it," (f) "I was afraid I would be rejected," and (g) "A condom reduces the emotional closeness." For each reason, they answered, "often," "sometimes," "rarely," or "never."

## Residence History

Men also described their residence history using one of four options: always lived in the same area or community that you live now; lived in the area, moved away to another small town or rural area, then moved back; lived in the area, moved to a city, and then came back to the area; and, lived in a city most of your life and moved to the area that you live now. For the purposes of analyses men were divided into two groups, those who had always lived in a rural area and those who had lived in an urban area at some time.

# Results

## *Personal Characteristics*

The levels of education reported by the men varied. Eleven percent had only completed high school, 25% completed trade or technical school, 28% had taken some college courses, 24% had completed college, and 10% had advanced degrees. The men reported the following monthly incomes: 7% less than $500, 15% from $501–999, 37% from $1000–1999, 24% from $2000–2999, 7% from $3000–3999, and 9% $4000 and over. Over half (54%, $n = 49$) of the men had always lived in a rural area and the rest of the men (46%, $n = 41$) had lived in an urban area at some point. Based on the Kinsey-type scale, 65% said they were "completely gay," 21% said they were "almost totally gay, slightly heterosexual," 8% said they were "mostly gay, more than slightly heterosexual," 4% said they were "equally gay and heterosexual," and, 2% said they were "almost totally heterosexual, but slightly gay."

## *Relationship Status*

Almost half (46%, $n = 45$) were in long term relationships that had lasted at least six months. Two men lived with women, and the others in relationships lived with men. Many (83%, n = 29) couples lived together; only 6 couples maintained separate residences. Relationships ranged from one to thirty years in duration, with an average of about 10 years. When asked to describe their relationships, 85% said they were in a committed relationship, 10% said they were dating, and 5% said they were likely to become a committed couple.

## *Methods for Meeting Sexual Partners*

Many (42%) did not answer the question about where they met sexual partners because they had sex with their primary partner only (34%), or had no sexual partners in the last six months (8%). Of the sexually active single men, private parties, dance clubs, or bars were the most common locales, all noted by about one-third of the men, and 18% met partners through mutual friends. Only 14% of the entire sample met men at public venues such as parks and rest stops, and the same number met other men using Internet chat-rooms. Very few met other men in adult bookstores (two men), at gay-oriented campgrounds (two men), or in sex clubs (one man). Only four men met other sexual partners at work.

## Sexual Partners

In reporting about their current relationship, of the 45 men in relationships, half (49%) had other sexual partners. As to their partners, more than half (56%) of the men said their partners had extra-relationship partners, 5% (2 men) said their partners did not have other sexual partners, and over one-third (39%) did not know about partners' other sexual experiences. In only five cases did the respondent acknowledge other partners as well as knowing that his partner had other sexual partners; thus, there were few "open relationships." The more frequent occurrence, reported by 35% of the men, was that the respondents had other sexual partners but did not know if their partners did.

In terms of types of partners, 10% of the entire sample reported no sexual partners in the last six months; 64% reported primary partners; 44% reported casual partners; and, 36% reported unknown or anonymous partners. (These categories are not mutually exclusive.) Of those with sexual partners, three-quarters with primary partners had one partner, and one-quarter had more than one primary partner. For those reporting casual partners, 30% had one casual partner, 68% had from two to five, and one man had from six to ten casual partners in the last six months. Of those men having unknown partners, 28% had one such partner, 56% reported from two to five, and 8% reported six to ten partners. Two men said they had 11 to 50 casual sexual partners, and one man reported more than 50. Of men with primary partners, 3% had HIV positive partners; 77% had partners known to be HIV negative; and, 20% did not know the HIV status of their primary partners. Of those with casual partners, 5% had HIV+ partners, 51% had HIV negative partners; and, 44% did not know the HIV status of their casual partners. Of the men who had sex with unknown partners in the last six months, one man knew his partner was HIV positive. Only 16% of men with unknown sexual partners knew these partners were HIV negative. Most men with unknown partners (81% or 30 men) were unaware of partners' HIV status.

Seven percent of the men reported ever having a sexual partner known to be HIV positive. Two men had two such partners; one reported six HIV positive partners; one reported ten HIV positive partners; and, one man said he had 25 sexual partners who were HIV positive.

## Sexual Risk Behavior

The sexual behavior the men reported with different kinds of partners over the last six months is depicted in Table 1. Over one-third (36%) reported no receptive anal intercourse. One third (37%) engaged in receptive anal intercourse but did not always use condoms, and 16% always used condoms when having receptive anal intercourse. About half of the men with primary partners did not always use condoms in unprotected receptive anal intercourse. Men who were in a relationship and had outside sexual partners ($M = 2.48$, $SD = .93$) were more likely to have unprotected receptive anal sex with primary partners than single men ($M = 1.79$, $SD = .90$), $t(61) = 2.85$, $p < .01$, a moderate effect, $d = .75$. Of men with casual partners, only 13% reported not always using condoms when having receptive anal intercourse. Of the men who had unknown partners, one-quarter did not always use condoms in receptive anal intercourse.

There were differences in the patterns of condom use for receptive anal sex between men who had always lived in a rural area and men who had lived in an urban area at some time. More of the men who had lived in a rural area their entire life (42%, $n = 20$) engaged in unprotected receptive anal sex than men who had lived in an urban area at some point (17%, $n = 7$), $\chi^2 (1, N = 89) = 6.33$, $p < .05$. Men who had always lived in a rural area also reported having more partners (M = .54, $SD = .71$) with whom they had unprotected receptive anal sex than men who had lived urban areas (M = .17, $SD = .38$), $t(74) = 3.12$, $p < .01$. This difference is considered a moderate effect, $d = .68$.

Using the Ostrow et al. (1998) risk categories, of the 96 men for whom all the needed data were available, 22% were at no risk for HIV infection, 30% were at low risk, 26% were at modified high risk; and, 22% were at high risk for HIV infection. Analyses of variance were conducted comparing the four sets of men on the demographic information available. Only age yielded a significantly significant finding, $F(3, 92) = 3.30$, $p < .05$. Follow-up Scheffe tests found that the no risk group ($M = 42.67$, $SD = 10.14$) was significantly older than the modified high risk group ($M = 24.16$, $SD = 11.17$).

**Table 1**
*Sexual Behavior with Different Partner Types in the Past Six Months (N = 99)*

| Sexual Behavior | Total | | Types of Sexual Partner | | | | | |
|---|---|---|---|---|---|---|---|---|
| | N | % | Primary $n = 65$ | | Casual $n = 45$ | | Unknown $n = 36$ | |
| No sexual behavior | 10 | 10.3 | | | | | | |
| No receptive anal intercourse | 35 | 36.1 | | | | | | |
| Receptive anal intercourse not always with condoms | 36 | 37.1 | 31 | 47.6 | 6 | 13.3 | 9 | 25.0 |
| Receptive anal intercourse always with condoms | 16 | 16.5 | 18 | 27.6 | 17 | 37.7 | 14 | 38.8 |

As to lifetime HIV positive partners with whom men reported unprotected receptive anal intercourse, 7% had unprotected anal sex with known HIV positive partners: two had one HIV positive partner, and one each had two, six, and ten partners. Most men (92%) did not report unprotected sex with HIV positive partners. Two men were HIV positive themselves, two men were HIV negative, and one man had never been tested for HIV.

## Personal and Interpersonal Strategies to Minimize Risk of HIV Infection

The activities single men and men in non-monogamous relationships used to minimize HIV risk are presented in Table 2. The most consistently used risk reduction strategies were avoiding receptive anal sex, avoiding alcohol and drug use during sex, asking about partners' HIV status, and discussing condom use with partners. However, nearly one-third (31%) did not avoid receptive anal sex, 24% never asked partners about HIV status, 36% never asked partners about their health, and 32% never discussed condom use. These men would be at risk for HIV infection if they had unprotected sex with HIV positive partners.

**Table 2**

*Frequency of HIV-Risk Reducing Sexual Behavior of Sexually Active Single Men and Men in Non-Monogamous Relationships (N = 99)*

| Sexual Behavior | Always | | Sometimes | | Never | |
|---|---|---|---|---|---|---|
| | n | % | n | % | N | % |
| Not receptive partner in anal intercourse | 14 | 27 | 22 | 42 | 16 | 31 |
| Not insertive partner in anal intercourse | 10 | 20 | 22 | 43 | 19 | 37 |
| Avoided contact with partner's semen | 10 | 19 | 37 | 70 | 6 | 11 |
| Avoided drugs and alcohol when having sex | 18 | 34 | 24 | 45 | 11 | 21 |
| Asked about partner's HIV status | 15 | 29 | 24 | 47 | 12 | 24 |
| Asked about partner's health history | 5 | 9 | 29 | 55 | 19 | 36 |
| Discussed condom use before sex | 12 | 23 | 24 | 45 | 17 | 32 |

Single men ($M = 2.18$, $SD = .81$) were more likely to discuss safe sex with new partners than men who were in relationships and had outside partners ($M = 1.70$, $SD = .64$), $t(58) = 2.33$, $p < .05$, a moderate effect, $d = .66$. When asked about topics men discussed before sex, the most common conversation was about unwillingness to have unprotected anal sex. Half (50%) had such conversations in the past six months. As to discussions men *never* had with sex partners, 37% said they never asked a new partner about condoms, 40% never inquired about a partner's sexual history, 70% never discussed HIV testing, 60% never asked about STD's, and 67% did not ask about injection drug use.

Nearly three-quarters (72% or 71 men) of the men had been tested for HIV. Fewer of the men who had always lived in a rural area (61%, $n = 30$) had been tested for HIV than men who had lived in an urban area at some time (83%, $n = 34$), $\chi^2 (1, N = 90) = 5.12$, $p < .05$. Of the men who had been tested, 19% had been tested once, 21% were tested twice, and 14% three times. More than one-quarter (27%) said they had been tested from four to nine times; and, 15% said from 10 to 15 times. Three men (3%) had been tested more than fifteen times (20, 24, and 25 HIV tests).

Of the 70 men reporting an HIV test, four said their last HIV test was positive, and the rest reported negative results. Of the men who had been tested, 67% expected to be tested in the future, 21% said they might be tested, and the rest (12% or 8 men) did not expect further testing. Men who had not been tested commonly gave two reasons. Half (50%) said they were at low risk for HIV infection, and 21% said they would be afraid to learn test results. One man said he feared needles; one said he had no health insurance; and, one had not had a sexual experience with another man. Of those men who were at highest risk by engaging in unprotected anal sex with a known HIV positive partner, all had been tested for HIV except one man who said that he would be afraid to learn the results.

## Intoxication During Sexual Activity

Men more often reported more use of drugs or alcohol during the last six months with unknown or casual partners than with primary partners. Whereas only 12% reported having one drink with a primary partner, 33% did so with casual partners, and 45% with anonymous partners. Over half (55%) reported two drinks with anonymous partners, compared to 48% and 44% for primary and casual partners respectively. As to more than five drinks, 40% did this with primary partners, 23% with casual partners, and no men had more than five drinks with anonymous partners. Few reported drug or popper use. Eight men reported drug use with primary partners, five used drugs with casual partners, and three used drugs with anonymous partners. Seven men used poppers with primary partners, eight with casual partners, and ten with anonymous partners.

With regard to drug use leading to sexual behavior that was later regretted, most (83%) who reported any drug use said they never regretted any behavior, 15% said they occasionally regretted their behavior, and 2% often had regrets. In an answer to an open-ended question that asked whether or not participants had done something sexual that they had regretted after using drugs or alcohol, one man wrote "I had a few drinks at a bar, and tricked. I probably wouldn't have tricked if I hadn't had those drinks." Most men who provided comments to the same statement noted the impairment of their judgment due to excessive alcohol consumption.

## *Assessment of Personal Risk of HIV Infection*

Most men felt they were at much less likely to get AIDS than "the average gay or bisexual man." Nearly half (45%) said they were much less likely; 24% said a little less likely, and 25% said their risk was similar to the average gay or bisexual man. Single men rated their chances of getting HIV as higher ($M = 2.17$, $SD = 1.06$) than men who were in relationships and had outside sexual partners ($M = 1.57$, $SD = .75$), $t(61) = 2.30$, $p < .05$, a moderate effect, $d = .66$. Three men felt they were a little more likely to get AIDS, and three men said they were much more likely to get AIDS, than the average MSM. Correspondingly, on the related question of the riskiness of their sexual behavior, about half (46%) said their behavior was not at all risky, and only one man endorsed the "extremely risky" option. The rest rated themselves at or above values denoting little risk.

## Barriers to Avoiding Unprotected Receptive Anal Intercourse

Reasons given by men who had ever engaged in unprotected anal intercourse for not using condoms are shown in Table 3. The most frequently occurring reasons were fear of rejection, loss of emotional closeness, fear of offending a partner, and embarrassment. However, all seven reasons were at least sometimes involved in unprotected sex for more than three-quarters of the men, suggesting that several reasons simultaneously contribute to the situation. Indeed, Cronbach's alpha for these items was .83; showing consistency among the reasons men gave for engaging in unprotected anal sex.

**Table 3**
*Reasons Given for Not Using Condoms in Receptive Anal Intercourse (N = 99)*

| Reason | Often | | Sometimes | | Rarely | | Never | |
|---|---|---|---|---|---|---|---|---|
| | n | % | n | % | n | % | n | % |
| Partner would be offended | 54 | 72 | 13 | 17 | 6 | 8 | 2 | 3 |
| It would spoil the mood | 48 | 68 | 14 | 20 | 7 | 10 | 2 | 3 |
| It would reduce pleasure | 45 | 61 | 13 | 17 | 8 | 11 | 8 | 11 |
| It was too much trouble | 45 | 63 | 14 | 20 | 7 | 10 | 5 | 7 |
| I felt embarrassed | 52 | 70 | 14 | 19 | 4 | 5 | 4 | 5 |
| I was afraid I would be rejected | 56 | 76 | 8 | 11 | 7 | 9 | 3 | 4 |
| Condoms reduce emotional closeness | 52 | 73 | 8 | 11 | 6 | 8 | 5 | 7 |

## Discussion

This study was an exploratory attempt to describe the sexual behavior patterns of rural men who have sex with other men. The focus was on rural men's relationships, how they meet sexual partners, the types of partners they were involved with, and their sexual behavior with different kinds of partners. Particular attention was paid to behavior increasing risk of HIV infection, strategies men used to decrease their risk of exposure to HIV, and the relationship between alcohol and drug use and HIV risk. Despite the small sample, it was hoped results would lead to more extensive research linking characteristics of rural life with the life situations of men who have sex with men, some of whom identify as gay or bisexual, and some of whom do not.

We endeavored to describe the sexual activities of rural MSM, but there are few directly comparable urban data, so it is uncertain how much these men's rural residential status affects their sexual behavior. One comparison group are the MSM in the Urban Men's Health Study (Catania et al., 2001). A probability-based sample of four cities, the UMHS involved interviews with 2881 men in San Francisco, New York, Chicago, and Los Angeles. The sample ranges in age from 18 to over 80, with 37% in their 30s; two-thirds had at least a college degree or some post-graduate education, 21% were from racial and ethnic minority backgrounds, and nearly half of the men reported having a primary partner (Stall et al., 2001). In our sample, men ranged in age from 18 to 69. The average age was 38, and 37% were in their 30s. One-third had graduated from college or had advanced degrees. Only 5% were non-White. Whereas in the urban sample, 40% earned $40,000 or less and a quarter earned more than $80,000, only 9% of the rural men reported incomes over $48,000, 7% earned between $37,000 and $48,000, and the rest earned less. And, in this study, more than half (54%) had a partner. Although Stall, Hays, Waldo, Ekstrand, & McFarland (2000) did not provide prevalence figures on sexual behavior, rural MSM would have fewer opportunities for sexual contact with other men. Thus, rural men would, in general, be at less risk, partly because the probability of their having sex with an HIV+ man is lower than in urban areas: the prevalence rate for HIV infection was 17% in the UMHS. Also, in the rural areas sampled in this project, there are not the bathhouses or circuit parties (Binson et al., 2001; Mansergh et al., 2001; Mattison, Ross, Wolfson, &

Franklin 2001; Woods, Binson, Mayne, Gore, & Rebchook, 2001) that may be high risk sites for urban men. One-third of the rural MSM met sexual partners at private parties, dance clubs, and bars. Few met other men in public places (such as parks or rest stops) or through Internet chat-rooms. Thus, the men in the rural sample had lower incomes and educational levels, were nearly all White, and had less access to high risk venues than did urban men (these differences make comparisons on sexual behavior between samples problematic as the groups do not differ only in urban vs. rural status).

Over half of the MSM in this study said they had receptive anal sex in the past six months. Of these men, 37% reported using a condom only some of the time. This percent is somewhat lower that the 27% of men Kelly et al. (1992) found to have engaged in unprotected intercourse in a two month period, but this figure was for men not in monogamous relationships and the data were collected some time ago. In our data, single men and men in open relationships had more sexual partners in the last six months than other men. More partnered men engaged in unprotected receptive anal intercourse than single men, consistent with other findings (e.g., Wagner, Remien, & Carballo-Dieguez, 2000). Although MSM appear to be well informed about HIV transmission, public health guidelines, and safer sex practices (Hospers & Kok, 1995), many do not consistently engage in low risk behavior, and alternate between high and low risk behavior. Some factors associated with high risk behavior are more sexual partners, affective fluctuations (e.g., self-esteem, depression, and loneliness), low perceived personal risk, the perception that precautionary changes are not normative, high reinforcement of past sexual behaviors, and a health locus of control associated with luck or fate (Hospers & Kok, 1995; Kelly et al., 1992; Stall et al., 2000). More recent work has also focused on childhood sexual abuse (Paul, Catania, Pollack, & Stall, 2001).

There are limitations of the study that need to be acknowledged. One concerns the representativeness of the sample. The difficulties of involving gay and bisexual men in research studies are well-known, even in urban areas (Blair, 1999). Meyer and Colten (1999) have shown that urban gay and bisexual men who volunteer for research projects are different from other gay and bisexual men living in the same geographical area. Increasingly, epidemiological research has endeavored to generate representative samples of MSM. Two approaches have been used. One approach involves research exclusively focused upon such men, and samples are drawn from neighborhoods within major metropolitan areas known to have high concentrations of gay and bisexual male residents (Paul et al., 2002). Other representative samples of MSM are extracted from survey research designed to answer research questions unrelated to sexual orientation. In such studies, sub samples of MSM, or men who self-identify as gay or bisexual, can be created if socio-demographic questions about same-sex sexual behavior or sexual identity have been asked. Such studies have accumulated in the last few years, including the use of major data-sets on adolescence (e.g., Russell & Joyner, 2001). No study using either approach has focused on rural MSM. Indeed, the first strategy could not be implemented in rural settings.

The strategies used to obtain the sample in this study were driven by the difficulties in identifying MSM in rural communities, and engaging them in participating in research. We worked through informal social networks of men, and involved men who were open enough about themselves to attend social events for gay and bisexual men, or who were willing to visit the small gay bars located in the large rural area that was the focus of the study. We cannot know how representative these men might be of other rural MSM.

## Implications for Intervention

The study's limitations notwithstanding, there are important implications to be drawn from our findings. Most basically, it is clear that prevention efforts in rural areas directed at MSM need to increase. Both single men and men in committed relationships should be targeted, as risky sexual behavior was not confined to monogamous couples. Half of the men in relationships reported other sexual partners, but many did not know if their partners were acting in a similar way. Nearly half of men reported casual partners and about a third reported anonymous partners in the last six months. More important than the number of partners are MSM's sexual practices. Many did not know the HIV status of their sexual partners. For men with casual partners, for instance, 44% did not know of their partners' status; of these, 13% did not always use condoms in receptive anal intercourse. Of those with anonymous partners, most did not know partners' statuses, yet one-quarter of these men did not consistently use condoms in receptive anal intercourse. The combination of multiple sexual partners, lack of knowledge of partners' HIV status, and risky sexual behavior is a pattern with an elevated probability of HIV infection, especially in areas with high HIV prevalence rates. It is in the latter that rural MSM may have a "protective factor," as HIV prevalence in rural communities among MSM is considerably lower than among urban MSM.

Despite these characteristics of their sexual behavior, very few MSM considered themselves at serious risk for HIV infection. For instance, most felt their activities were not risky at all, or put them at little risk. Yet, our category system for risk placed 30% at some risk and 22% at high risk, mostly as a result of unprotected receptive anal intercourse. While it is possible that the Ostrow et al. (1998) classification system produces false positives in terms of risk, it must be considered that these MSM may have minimized their evaluation of risk to avoid discomfort or to face pressure to modify their behavior. Certainly, our data about risk reduction strategies provide some indication of discomfort in adopting safer sex practices, with many showing reluctance to discuss condom use. On a more positive note, many lowered their risk of minimizing receptive anal sex, avoiding intoxication during sex, and discussing condom use. Further, many men had been tested for HIV, an encouraging finding given the importance of early identification and prophylactic medical intervention.

Professionals working with rural MSM must first exhibit gay-affirming attitudes and behaviors. This is crucial to the discussion of intimate aspects of their relationship situation and their sexual behavior. Detailed discussion of the sexual practices of men in couples (making no assumption of monogamy and no judgment as to its value) and of single men (making no assumptions about the value of multiple partners of different types) needs to occur to help men more accurately assess their risk. Methods for resisting unsafe practices and negotiating cautious sexual behavior need to be delineated. And, the degree to which risky behavior might be related to living in a rural community is another important focus. Such assessments can be incorporated into individual consultations with rural MSM, and they must also be part of prevention programming. Additionally, the use of the Internet as a vehicle for meeting sexual partners should be considered. As Stall et al. (2000) have noted, interactions "chat-rooms" provide opportunities to discuss safer sexual behavior (including inquiry into HIV status). Because rural MSM have fewer social opportunities to meet other men, this mode of meeting partners can be important in maintaining safer sex practices, and refusing contact with men who are unwilling to "be safe."

## Conclusions

The results of this exploratory study provide a preliminary glimpse into issues of sexual orientation for rural MSM, a group that has been understudied to date. Several earlier studies reported that gay and bisexual men in rural areas continued to engage in risky sexual behavior despite perceived risk (Bell et al., 1991; Berry, 2000; Cohn, 1997; Preston et al., 2004). Moreover, since HIV/AIDS originated primarily in large cities, urban gay communities have highly developed health and social service infrastructures that provide many educational programs and resources to support the maintenance of less risky behavior. In contrast, rural populations of gay and bisexual men are usually fragmented and disenfranchised, and have fewer educational and health care resources for HIV/AIDS at their disposal (Sowell & Christensen, 1996). On the other hand, HIV prevalence is considerably lower in rural communities.

An understanding of the rural context is necessary for a complete analysis of MSM sexual behavior patterns. We have argued elsewhere (Preston et al., 2002, 2004) that rural MSM's behavior and identities are influenced by often conflicting social determinants — the influence of their families and local communities, which tend to stigmatize same-sex sexual orientation, and the influence of gay friends and the connections they have to the larger "gay community," with which they affiliate despite its lack of local presence. Additional research with larger samples will be needed to delineate how living in a rural community influences the behavior — social as well as sexual — of men who have sex with men, whether or not they identify as gay or bisexual.

### NOTE

The authors give their sincere thanks to the men who participated in this research and to John G. Bell for his efforts in directing the project. Completion of this manuscript was facilitated by grant RO1-MH62981 from the National Institute of Mental Health to the first two authors. Correspondence should be addressed to Deborah Bray Preston, School of Nursing, College of Health and Human Development, The Pennsylvania State University, 205E Health and Human Development East, University Park, PA 16802. Electronic mail: dqp@psu.edu.

**REFERENCES**

Anderson, D. A., & Lane-Shaw, S. (1994). Starting a support group for families and partners of people with HIV/AIDS in a rural setting. *Social Work, 39*(1), 135–138.

Bell, A. P., Weinberg, M. S., & Hammersmith, S. K. (1991). *Sexual preference: Its development in men and women.* Bloomington: Indiana University.

Berry, D. E. (2000). Rural acquired immunodeficiency syndrome in low and high prevalence areas. *Southern Medical Journal, 93,* 36–43.

Binson, D., Woods, W. J., Pollack, L., Paul, J., Stall, R., & Catania, J. A. (2001). Differential HIV risk in bathhouses and public cruising areas. *American Journal of Public Health, 91,* 1482–1486.

Blair, J. (1999). A probability sample of urban gay males: The use of two-phase adaptive sampling. *The Journal of Sex Research, 36,* 39–44.

Catania, J. A., Osmond, D., Stall, R., Pollack, L., Paul, J. P., Blower, S. et al. (2001). The continuing HIV epidemic among men who have sex with men. *American Journal of Public Health, 91,* 907–914.

Center for Rural Pennsylvania. (2001). Pennsylvania Data Base: Harrisburg, PA.

Centers for Disease Control and Prevention (2001). *HIV prevention strategic plan through 2005.* Retrieved July 12, 2002 http://www.cdc.gov/nchstp/od/hiv_plan/default.htm

Cohn, S. E. (1997). AIDS in rural America. *Journal of Rural Health, 13,* 237–239.

D'Augelli, A. R., & Hart, M. M. (1987). Gay women, men, and families in rural communities: Toward the development of helping communities. *American Journal of Community Psychology, 13,* 79–93.

D'Augelli, A. R., Hart, M. M., & Collins, C. (1987). Social support patterns in a rural network of lesbian women. *Journal of Rural Community Psychology, 8,* 12–22.

D'Augelli, A. R., Preston, D. B., Kassab, C. D., & Cain, R. E. (2002). Rural men who have sex with men: An exploratory study of sexual orientation characteristics and adjustment patterns. *Journal of Rural Community Psychology,* [Electronic version] *5*(2).

Garnets, L. D., & D'Augelli, A. R. (1994). Empowering lesbian and gay communities: A call for collaboration with community psychology. *American Journal of Community Psychology, 22,* 447–470.

Herek, G. M., Cogan, J. C., Gillis, J. R., & Glunt, E. K. (1998). Correlates of internalized homophobia in a community sample of lesbians and gay men. *Journal of the Gay and Lesbian Medical Association, 2,* 17–25.

Hospers, H. J., & Kok, G. (1995). Determinants of safe and risk-taking sexual behavior among gay men: A review. *AIDS Education and Prevention, 7,* 74–96.

Kelly, J. A., Murphy, D. A., Roffman, R. A., Solomon, L. J., Winett, R. A., Stevenson, L. Y., et al. (1992). Acquired immunodeficiency syndrome/human immunodeficiency virus risk behavior among gay men in small cities. Findings of a 16-city national sample. *Archives of Internal Medicine, 152,* 2293–2297.

Kus, R. J., & Smith, G. B. (1995). Referrals and resources for chemically dependent gay and lesbian clients. *Journal of Gay and Lesbian Social Services, 2,* 91–107.

Laumann, E. O., Gagnon, J. H., Michael, R. T., & Michaels, S. (1994). *The social organization of sexuality: Sexual practices in the United States.* Chicago: University of Chicago.

Lindhorst, T. (1997). Lesbians and gay men in the country: Practice implications for rural social workers. In J. D. Smith & R. J. Mancoske (Eds.), *Rural gays and lesbians: Building on the strengths of communities* (pp. 1–11). New York: Haworth.

Mancoske, R. J. (1997). Rural HIV/AIDS social services for gays and lesbians. In J. D. Smith & R. J. Mancoske (Eds.), *Rural gays and lesbians: Building on the strengths of communities* (pp. 37–52). New York: Haworth.

Mansergh, G., Colfax, G. M., Marks, G., Rader, M., Guzman, R., & Buchbinder, S. (2001). The Circuit Party Men's Health Survey: Findings and implications for gay and bisexual men. *American Journal of Public Health, 91,* 953–958.

Martinez-Brawley, E. E., & Blundall, J. (1989). Farm families' preferences toward personal social services. *Social Work, 34,* 513–522.

Mattison, A. M., Ross, M. W., Wolfson, T., & Franklin, D. (2001). Circuit party attendance, club drug use, and unsafe sex in gay men. *Journal of Substance Abuse, 13,* 119–126.

Mayne T. J., & O'Leary, A. (1993). Family support is more important than friend or partner support in reducing distress among suburban and rural gay men. *Proceedings of the International Conference on AIDS, 9,* 120.

Meyer, I. H., & Colten, M. (1999). Sampling gay men: Random digit dialing versus sources in the community. *Journal of Homosexuality, 37,* 99–110.

Ostrow, D. G., DiFranceisco, W., & Wagstaff, D. (1998). The coping and change study of men at risk of AIDS: Sexual Behavior and Behavior Change Questionnaire. In C. M. Davis, W. L. Yarber, R. Bauserman, G. Sheer, & L. Davis (Eds.), *Handbook of sexuality-related measures* (pp. 547–553). Thousand Oaks, CA: Sage.

Paul, J. P., Catania, J., Pollack, L., Moshowitz, J., Canchola, J., Mills, T., et al. (2002). Suicide attempts among gay and bisexual men: Lifetime prevalence and antecedents. *American Journal of American Public Health, 92,* 1338–1345.

Paul, J. J., Catania, J., Pollack, L., & Stall, R. (2001). Understanding childhood sexual abuse as a predictor of sexual risk-taking among men who have sex with men: The Urban Men's Health Study. *Child Abuse and Neglect, 25,* 557–584.

Preston, D. B., D'Augelli, A. R., Cain, R. E., & Schulze, F. W. (2002). Issues in the development of HIV-preventive interventions for men who have sex with men (MSM) in rural areas. *Journal of Primary Prevention 23,* 201–216.

Preston, D. B., D'Augelli, A. R., Kassab, C. D., Cain, R. E., & Schulze, F. W. & Starks, M. T. (2004). The influence of stigma on the sexual risk behavior of rural men who have sex with men. *AIDS Education and Prevention, 16*(4), 291–303.

Russell, S. T., & Joyner, K. (2001). Adolescent sexual orientation and suicide risk: Evidence from a national study. *American Journal of Public Health, 91,* 1276–1281.

Schur, C. L., Berk, M. L., Dunbar, J. R., Shapiro, M. F., Cohn, S. E., & Bozzette, S. A. (2002). Where to seek care: An examination of people in rural areas with HIV/AIDS. *Journal of Rural Health 18*(2), 337–347.

Shidlo, A. (1994). Internalized homophobia: Conceptual and empirical issues in measurement. In B. Greene & G. M. Herek (Eds.), *Lesbian and gay psychology: Theory, research, and clinical applications* (pp. 176–205). Thousand Oaks, CA: Sage.

Smith, J. D. (1997). Working with larger systems: Rural lesbians and gays. In J. D. Smith & R. J. Mancoske (Eds.), *Rural gays and lesbians: Building on the strengths of communities* (pp. 37–52). New York: Haworth.

Sowell, R., & Christensen, P. (1996). HIV infection in rural communities. *Nursing Clinics of North America, 31,* 107–123.

Stall, R., Hays, R. B., Waldo, C. R., Ekstrand, M., & McFarland, W. (2000). The gay '90s: A review of research in the 1990's on sexual behavior and HIV risk among men who have sex with men. *AIDS, 14* (Suppl. 3), S101–S114.

Stall, R., Paul, J. P., Greenwood, G., Pollack, L. M., Bein, E., Crosby, C. M., Mills, T. C., et al, (2001). Alcohol use, drug use, and alcohol-related problems among men who have sex with men: The Urban Men's Health Study. *Addiction, 96,* 1589–1601.

Wagner, G. J., Remien, R. H., & Carballo-Dieguez, A. (2000). Prevalence of extradyadic sex in male couples of mixed HIV status and its relationship to psychological distress and relationship quality. *Journal of Homosexuality, 39*(2), 31–46.

Weitz, R. (1991). *Life with AIDS.* New Brunswick, NJ: Rutgers University.

Woods, W. J., Binson, D., Mayne, T. J., Gore, L. R., & Rebchook, G. M. (2001). Facilities and HIV prevention in bathhouse and sex club environments. *Journal of Sex Research, 38,* 68–74.

*Chapter 11*

# Measurement in Rural Research:
## Matching the Instrument to the Population

### JANET AMBROGNE SOBCZAK

## Introduction

The value of any research endeavor rests on the foundation of appropriate measurement (Switzer, Wisniewski, Belle, Dew, & Schultz, 1999). Measurement is achieved through the use of instruments. Because instruments are developed with particular populations, they are subject to culture-bound assumptions. People from a different background than the one for which the instrument was developed may use, define or interpret the meanings of words and phrases differently (Strickland, 1998). Consequently, the quality of the data may be compromised due to under-endorsement or over-endorsement of items, biases related to certain items, and different interpretations of the items (Switzer et al.). Therefore, it is critical to consider the characteristics of the population of interest in all measurement decisions.

Despite obvious importance, comparatively less attention has been given to this aspect of instrumentation. As Strickland (1998) noted, the demonstrated psychometric soundness of an instrument can easily overshadow the more practical issues related to the use of that instrument with a particular population. However, even the most reliable and valid instruments may perform differently when administered to a new population, or in a different setting. The purpose of this paper is to discuss issues related to instrument selection for rural populations. Few instruments have been developed specifically for rural populations (Fahs, Findholt & Daniel, 2003). Consequently, instruments used in rural research may have limited validity and reliability. Attention to the fit between an instrument and the characteristics of the population under study will hopefully lead to the increased use of culturally appropriate and psychometrically sound instruments in rural studies.

## Knowing the Cultural Geography

Spradley (1980) defined culture as "... the acquired knowledge people use to interpret experience and generate behavior" (p. 6). Culture encompasses beliefs, practices, customs, values, knowledge and attitudes that are impacted by the environment and assimilated through social networks and community norms (Patrick, Stein, Porta, Porter & Rickets, 1988; Spector, 1991; Switzer et al., 1999). Rural dwellers have a different cultural background from their urban, suburban and even frontier counterparts. These differences may impact how they interpret and respond to items on instruments developed and used in these other populations.

Terms such as "rural culture" and "rural dwellers" do not imply one homogenous group. Rural people share the commonality of living in a rural area. However, values, beliefs, customs, norms, demographics, geography and other environmental factors may vary from one rural locale to another (Slama, 2004). One cannot assume that an instrument that performs well in an urban setting will perform equally well in a rural setting. Nor can the assumption be made that an instrument with good reliability and validity in one rural setting will yield equally solid psychometrics in another. Sound decisions about instrumentation begin with a foundation of knowledge about the specific rural population under study, or as Slama (2004) coined "Knowing your cultural geography" (p. 9). Questions such as "What are the characteristics of my population?" "How does my study population differ from urban, suburban and frontier populations?" and "How does my population differ from other rural locales?" are wise to pose prior to instrument selection. The answers to such questions will be invaluable in deciding whether to use an existing instrument as is, adapt an existing instrument, or develop a new instrument.

## Existing Instruments

There is certainly a need for new instruments that have been developed and tested with rural populations. However, prior to taking on the time and labor intensive task of instrument development, it is wise to search for existing instruments that have potential for use in the study. There is little point in developing a new instrument if one is already available and appropriate for the study and the population of interest. Existing instruments can be classified as "established" and "new." According to Switzer et al. (1999), established instruments have been used in more than one research setting and have good reliability and validity estimates in each setting. An instrument that does not meet these criteria should be considered a new instrument.

It is ideal to use established instruments that are readily available, cost-effective, easy to administer, not overly taxing on either respondents or those administering the measures, have good widespread use, and good reliability and validity estimates. However, the appropriateness of an instrument for use in a study must first be determined. This entails evaluating the fit between the purpose and objectives of the study and specific properties of the instrument including: (a) the conceptual basis of the instrument; (b) the measurement approach and framework of the instrument; and (c) the results of psychometric testing.

### *Conceptual Basis*

The conceptual basis refers to what the instrument purports to measure. Terms such as concept, construct and even latent variable are often used interchangeably to refer to the abstract idea captured by an instrument. For simplicity, the term concept will be used in this paper. Instruments provide a means of translating an abstract concept into concrete observable psychosocial or physiological phenomena that can be consistently measured in a study sample (Waltz, Strickland & Lenz, 1991). Simply put, the foundation of any instrument is a concept.

Interpretations of a particular concept and the way in which that concept is defined can vary greatly by such characteristics as gender, ethnicity, age, occupation, education and geographic location

(Ferketich, Phillips, & Verran, 1993). It is necessary to first determine if the attributes of the concept measured by the instrument are congruent with the attributes of the concept being measured in the study population (Fahs et al., 2003). If, for example, one is looking at barriers to mental health care, it is first necessary to have some understanding of what may constitute barriers in the study population. Issues pertinent to a rural population such as a desire for anonymity, harvest season, or the lack of a paved route to the clinic may not be measured by items in an instrument developed with a sample of urban dwellers. In such a situation, it is prudent to consider the utility of the instrument in the study.

## *Measurement Type and Framework*

The type of measure and the measurement framework of an instrument should be appropriate for the questions and goals guiding the study. A quantitative approach, using numerical data to obtain information, is the best choice for studies stating hypotheses and/or posing questions best addressed with objective data. Scales, some questionnaires, tests and observational checklists are examples of such instruments. If subjective data are desired, a qualitative approach using instruments comprised of open-ended questions, sentence completion, narratives, structured or semi-structured interviews and structured or non-structured observations are more suitable.

The measurement framework refers to the standard used when comparing respondents' scores on a measure, and guides both the design and interpretation of most quantitative measures. If study goals include comparing the respondents with a comparison or norm group, it is best to use a well-established norm-referenced measure (Havens, 2001). Norm-referenced measures distribute subjects along a possible range of scores. Criterion-referenced measures are the better choice if goals of the study include determining if respondents have mastered a set of predetermined target behaviors (Waltz et al., 1991). When criterion-referenced measures are used, respondents are compared to a preset criterion rather than a group average (Turnbull, 1989).

## *Psychometric Testing*

Psychometric testing refers to reliability and validity estimates which are expressed as a matter of degree (Burns & Grove, 2001). An important consideration in selecting instruments is the results of previous psychometric testing. It is equally important to look at the characteristics of the study populations used with the instrument. Has the instrument been used with similar or different populations? Could differences between the populations influence how respondents answer items? What were the identified limitations of previous studies? Are there any anticipated problems using this instrument with a different population?

Reliability refers to the consistency of the measures obtained in an instrument in the areas of stability (test-retest reliability, inter-rater, intra-rater), equivalence (parallel forms reliability, split-half) and homogeneity (internal consistency reliability) (Burns & Grove, 2001). Reliability is typically expressed as a correlation coefficient with a range of 0 (no reliability) to 1.00 (perfect reliability). Nunnally and Bernstein (1994) have recommended 0.70 as the minimum acceptable reliability for a new instrument and 0.80 for established instruments. Critical physiological instruments may have a higher minimum acceptable level (Burns & Grove). While widely used, one criticism of correlation coefficients is that they denote an association between scores. Methods that score on actual agreement between scores such as intraclass correlation for continuous scales, Kendall's index for concordance for ordinal scales, and Cohen's kappa coefficient for dichotomous scales have gained increased prominence and are particularly useful with test-retest, inter-rater and intra-rater reliability (Switzer et al., 1999).

Validity is a determination of the extent to which the instrument actually reflects the underlying concept (Burns & Grove, 2001). In other words, does the instrument actually measure what it is supposed to measure in that specific group or setting? Three interrelated components of validity are: content validity, criterion validity and construct validity. Content validity addresses whether the individual items encompass the domains of the concept. Expert panels and focus groups of potential respondents are examples of strategies to establish content validity. Criterion validity is established by the extent to which the measure correlates with a very well established, or "gold standard" measure of the same concept and may be concurrent or predictive. Construct validity addresses how the instrument measures the underlying concept and tests hypothetical relationships between the concept and other variables. Methods to establish construct validity include contrasted groups, multi-trait-multi-method, and exploratory or confirmatory factor analysis (Burns & Grove; Switzer et al., 1999; Waltz et al., 1991).

While it is important to consider the results of psychometric testing, it is equally important to consider how reliability and validity estimates were obtained. For example, internal consistency reliability is one of the most popular ways of estimating reliability. However, this method is better suited for instruments developed from a norm-referenced framework, which is based on the theory of the Guassian curve (Switzer et al., 1999; Waltz et al., 1991). Test-retest reliability is well suited to physiological measures, but has more limitations with paper and pencil measures. Subjectively scored instruments are best evaluated using intra-rater and inter-rater reliability (Waltz et al.). Content validity is a prerequisite of instrument validity (Switzer, 1999). Therefore, content validity should always be assessed along with another type of validity and should not be considered a "stand-alone" validity estimate.

As a rule, reliability and validity should be estimated each time an instrument is used. For established instruments, Switzer et al. (1999) suggest a minimum of internal consistency reliability and analysis to confirm factor structure. However, methods to establish reliability and validity should be well suited to the instrument. New instruments and any instrument being used with a rural population for the first time should be pilot tested. A pilot test will not only provide preliminary reliability and validity estimates, but will also identify problems with the instrument that may not have been anticipated such as ambiguous directions, poorly worded items and issues related to administration and scoring.

## Adapting an Existing Instrument

Perhaps an established instrument that measures the concept of interest is located. However, the instrument has not been used in a rural population and certain aspects of the instrument are questionably suitable. For example, the reading level of the instrument may not be appropriate, or items may contain words or phrases that are not familiar to the population of interest. The instrument may contain items that are not relevant or conversely, lack items that address relevant issues. One practical option is to modify the instrument by changing some aspect of the instrument such as item wording, reading level or instrument length. A second option is to create a "hybrid" instrument (Switzer et al., 1999, p. 405) by either combining items from the instrument with newly created items, or by combining items from the instrument with those from one or more other established instruments.

Prior to using any existing instrument that is not public domain, permission from the instrument developer and/or copyright owner must be obtained. If an existing instrument is to be modified or used to create a hybrid, it is helpful to also provide the developer/ copyright owner with a rationale for the proposed changes and any anticipated changes in the performance of the instrument. Changes to an existing instrument can pose a number of threats to the reliability and validity. However, there is a lack of literature addressing issues pertaining to adapting instruments for other English-speaking cultures or subcultures (Harris, Belyea, Mishel and Germino, 2003). These issues will be addressed here along with two examples of instruments adapted for use by a different population.

## *Modified Instruments*

Common modifications to instruments include: (a) shortening the length; (b) changing the wording; and (c) changing the response categories. Switzer et al. (1999) noted advantages to modifying an existing instrument versus developing a new instrument including some assurance that (a) the items in the instrument operated as a unified measure in the past, and (b) the wording of the items has a demonstrated clarity. When a decision is made to modify an instrument it is important to articulate a detailed rationale for the modifications to be made. This should include an adequate description of the original measure, steps taken to alter the measure, and any anticipated differences in the performance of the measure (Switzer, et al.).

In their study of how older, Southern Caucasian and African-American men and women manage uncertainty during treatment for cancer, Harris et al. (2003) provide an excellent example of how instruments can be modified for a different population. Preliminary qualitative work comprised of focus groups and individual interviews with members of the study population helped the authors identify necessary revisions. For example, the Symptom Intensity Scale (Moinpour, Hayden, Thompson, Feigi, & Metch, 1990 cited in Harris et al., 2003) was used to measure the intensity of side effects from cancer treatment. An item on this scale reading, "I seldom, if ever, have nausea" was changed to "I never have to throw-up" (p. 48) because the authors had learned that the phrase "have to throw up" was consistently used to describe "nausea." On the Management of Uncertainty in Illness Scale (Mishel & Braden, 1988 cited in Harris et al., 2003), and item reading, "The explanations they give me about my conditions seem hazy to me" was changed to "I do not understand what they have told me about my illness" (p. 47). By knowing the cultural geography, the authors had a sound rationale for changing approximately 50% of the total items of the scales used in their study to better reflect the jargon used by the study population.

Modified instruments should be pilot tested for preliminary reliability and validity estimates. With extensive modifications, it is wise to use more than one method to establish reliability. Content validity should always be established. If the length of the instrument has been shortened, factor analysis is necessary to evaluate the internal factor structure. When wording is changed, construct validity is necessary to determine if the measure still supports anticipated theoretical relationships (Switzer et al., 1999). In the above example, interrater and internal consistency reliability were used with correlation coefficients ranging from 0.63–0.93 (Harris et al., 2003). A team of nurses expert in caring for the population reviewed the modified instruments. The instruments were also pre-tested with 15 individuals representative of the sample to elicit feedback on the understandability of the instruments and the appropriateness of the terms used in the revisions. No specific methods were employed to establish construct validity. Rather, the authors used the coefficient alphas as support that the instruments were measuring the intended concepts in all but one instrument.

## *Hybrid Instruments*

Hybrid instruments are developed by combining items from more than one established scale, or by combining newly created items with items from an established scale (Switzer et al., 1999). Hybrid instruments are most appropriate when existing scales do not adequately measure all the issues of interest and/or have questionable psychometric soundness. By creating a composite instrument, there is some assurance that the items from a well-established scale have been previously evaluated for clarity. Hybrid measures should be accompanied by a rationale that includes a description of the original measure(s), identified inadequacies in the original measure(s) that led to the creation of the hybrid, steps taken in item selection/creation, modifications to item stems and response categories and an explanation of how the hybrid measure is expected to respond differently from the original measure(s) (Switzer et al., 1999).

Compared to modified measures, hybrid measures are further removed from the original measure and are subject to more extensive testing (Switzer et al., 1999). Preliminary analysis including item distributions, inter-item and item-scale correlations and factor analysis is integral in decisions related to item retention and scale development. Ideally, reliability should be established in more than one way. Content validity will most likely have been addressed in the justifications for the hybrid. However, construct validity and possibly criterion validity are recommended (Switzer et al.).

An example of a hybrid measure is a survey that was developed for a rural population (Morgan, Fahs, & Klesh, 2005). The authors replicated a study of public attitudes regarding willingness to participate in medical research studies (Trauth, Musa, Siminoff, Jewell, & Ricci, 2000 cited in Morgan et al.). However, the purpose of the later study was to examine barriers to research participation of rural people from the more global perspective of health care research.

A hybrid measure was created by rewording items from the original measure and combining them with newly created items that addressed potential barriers to research participation by rural people. A review of literature and hypothesized rural influences provided the rationale for the rewording and added questions The end result was a 100-item survey with scales for willingness, knowledge, attitudes and barriers that was appropriate for the study goals and population. On the barriers scale, internal consistency and factor analysis were used to establish reliability and validity and the authors reported a Cronbach's alpha of 0.81 (see the following chapter for full report).

# Conclusion

Rural researchers are challenged by an overall lack of instruments developed for rural populations. Decisions regarding whether to use an existing instrument as is, adapt an instrument, or develop a new instrument are best made on a solid foundation of knowledge about the population under study. Examining the fit between the properties of the instrument, the goals of the study and the characteristics of the population of interest will provide the best chances of using instruments that are culturally appropriate, reliable and valid.

## REFERENCES

Burns, N., & Grove, S. K. (2001). *The practice of nursing research: Conduct, critique, & Utilization* (4th ed.). Philadelphia, PA: Saunders.

Fahs, P. S., Findholt, N., & Daniel, S. D. (2003). Themes and issues in rural nursing research. In M. S. Collins (Ed.), *Teaching / learning activities for rural community-based nursing practice* (pp. 156–172). Binghamton, NY: Decker School of Nursing, Binghamton University.

Ferketich, S., Phillips, L., & Verran, J. (1993). Development and administration of a survey instrument for cross-cultural research. *Research in Nursing and Health, 16*, 227–230.

Harris, L., Belyea, M., Mishel, M., & Germino, B. (2003). Issues in revising research instruments for use with southern populations. *Journal of National Black Nurses Association, 14*(2), 44–50.

Havens, G. A. D. (2001). A practical approach to the process of measurement in nursing. *Clinical Nurse Specialist, 15*(4), 146–152.

Morgan, L. L., Fahs, P. S., & Klesh, J. (2005). Barriers to research participation identified by rural people. *Journal of Agricultural Safety and Health, 11*(4), 407–414.

Nunnally, J. C., & Bernstein, I. H. (1994). *Psychometric theory* (3rd ed.). New York: McGraw-Hill.

Patrick, D. L., Stein, J., Poerta, M., Porter, C. Q., & Ricketts, T. C. (1988). Poverty, health service and health status in rural America. *The Milbank Quarterly, 66*, 105–136.

Slama, K. (2004). Rural culture is a diversity issue. Minnesota Psychologist (January). Retrieved January 26, 2006, from ttp://www.apa.org/rural/Rural_Culture_is_a_Diversity_Issue.pdf

Spradley, J. P. (1980). *Participant observation*. Fort Worth, TX: Harcourt Brace Jovanovich.

Strickland, O. L. (1998). Practical measurement. *Journal of Nursing Measurement, 6*(2), 107–109.

Switzer, G. E., Wisniewski, S. R., Belle, S. H., Dew, M. A., & Schultz, R. (1999). Selecting, developing, and evaluating research instruments. *Social Psychiatry and Psychiatric Epidemiology, 34,* 399–409.

Turnbull, J. M. (1989). What is ... normative versus criterion-referenced assessment. *Medical Teacher, 11*(2), 145–150.

Waltz, C. F., Strickland, O. L., & Lenz, E. R. (1991). *Measurement in nursing research* (2nd ed.), Philadelphia: F. A. Davis.

*Chapter 12*

# Barriers to Research Participation Identified by Rural People

### LINDSAY LAKE MORGAN, PAMELA STEWART FAHS, AND JAMIE KLESH

**Abstract:** It has been suggested anecdotally that rural people are less receptive to participating in research than other populations. Proposed reasons include culture, knowledge, attitudes, and barriers. Barriers to health care may also be barriers to research participation. A random sample of 5,000 households from a sampling frame of 45,000 property owners in a rural upstate New York county was selected. This article is a report of development of a Barriers scale from the findings of 865 completed surveys. The survey in this study contained 100 questions and was adapted from a pre-existing survey of public attitudes regarding willingness to participate in medical research. Factor analysis was utilized to isolate a Barriers to Participation in Research scale. Comparison of demographics and perceived barriers to participation were completed. Those who were classified as younger than the median sample age and male scored significantly lower on the barriers scale indicating more barriers to participation in health care research. Those with the highest perception of barriers were among the least willing to participate as research subjects. The findings inform assumptions researchers make about barriers to research and strategies are suggested to remove such barriers. Opening the doors to inclusion of rural people in health research studies will ultimately result in improved individual and community health in rural places.

Investigators committed to the inclusion of vulnerable and underrepresented populations in research have hypothesized about the barriers to participation of rural populations (Fahs, Findholt, & Daniel, 2003; Shreffler, 1999). Research participation of this group can have the outcome of building a research base that is more representative of the population as a whole, with the ultimate goal of improved health care quality.

The purpose of this study was to conduct a systematic replication of a study by Trauth et al. (Trauth, Musa, Siminoff, Jewell, & Ricci, 2000) and thus to further develop an instrument appropriate for use in rural populations. Systematic replication entails a significant modification of the design in order to increase empirical generalization (Beck, 1994). Trauth et al. (2000) studied public attitudes regarding willingness to participate in medical research studies. Questions on the survey in the present study went beyond medical research or clinical trials and examined barriers to participation in a more global category of health care research. In addition, because health care research is conducted by members of many disciplines, the survey included questions regarding barriers to participation in studies conducted by a range of health care providers, including doctors, nurses, social workers, and the more general term "scientists." Using an adaptation of the Trauth et al. (2000) survey and different procedures, a rural sample was surveyed to examine rural people's perceptions of scientific health care research.

The conceptualized relationships guiding this study proposed that rural dwellers' willingness to participate in research is affected by knowledge, attitudes, and barriers. Barriers to research have rural features such as access, driving conditions, lack of resources, and outsider status of the researcher.

## Review of the Literature

According to a public opinion poll conducted by Research!America (2003), Americans value information gained from scientific research. Research!America (Research!America, 2003) found that 78% of those polled believe that the United States should remain a leader in scientific research. Ninety-seven percent said that clinical research is of great or some value, and 63% stated that they would participate in a clinical research study. Respondents stated that the following would be a major concerns affecting participation: (1) reputation of institution, 76%; (2) improve the health of self/others, 69%; (3) privacy and confidentiality, 66%; (4) their physician's recommendations, 54%; and (5) incentives to participate, 14%. Interestingly, in this survey (Research!America, 2003) people trusted nurses (95%), pharmacists (94%), their physician (93%), medical schools and teaching hospitals (92%), and their dentists (90%) most for accurate research information.

Much of the literature on willingness to participate in research dwells on the acquisition of subjects for clinical or randomized controlled trials, which are the gold standard of medical research. Lovato et al. (Lovato, Hill, Hertert, Hunninghake, & Probstfield, 1997) reported on a systematic review of the literature on recruitment into clinical trials that covered published literature on the topic through 1995. This search identified over 4,000 titles and resulted in the annotation of 91 articles on subjects in medical research. These authors identified only 10 articles that related to barriers to participation in research within their review. Most reports from the late 1990s and first half of the following decade that have to do with willingness to participate in research can be broken down into four general categories. These include attitudes regarding participation (Corbie-Smith, Thomas, Williams, & Moody-Ayers, 1999; Ellis, 2000; Fallowfield et al., 1998; Fallowfield, L, Ratcliffe, & Souhami, 1997; Madsen et al., 2002; Norman et al., 1998; Trauth et al., 2000; Unson, Dunbar, Curry, Kenyon, & Prestwood, 2001), knowledge of subjects regarding participation (Apolone & Mosconi, 2003; Shavers, Lynch, & Burmeister, 2000b; Unson et al., 2001), barriers to participation (Daly et al., 2002; Ellis, Butow, Simes, Tattersall, & Dunn, 1999; Grunfeld, Zitzelsberger, Coristine, & Aspelund, 2002; Mouton, Harris, Rovi, Solorzano, & Johnson, 1997; Ross et al., 1999) and the effect of ethnicity or race on participation in research (Corbie-Smith et al., 1999; Fisher & Ball, 2003; Halpern et al., 2003; Harris, Gorelick, Samuels, & Bempong, 1996; Kennedy & Burnett, 2002; Outlaw, Bourjolly, & Barg, 2000; Shavers-Hornaday, Lynch, Burmeister, & Torner, 1997; Shavers, Lynch, & Burmeister, 2000a; Unson et al., 2001). Only a few studies have dealt with the issues of rural dwellers and their participation in research (Maurer et al., 2001; Norman et al., 1998; Pierce & Scherra, 2004; Powe & Weinrich, 1999; Shreffler, 1999).

Rural issues affecting research participation found in the literature included environmental barriers, cultural sensitivity, and knowledge. Pierce and Scherra (2004) discussed issues related to environmental barriers of isolation, weather, and distances traveled by the researcher in order to collect data in the homes of rural women. These authors reported on the trust evident in the visits with the subjects in their homes and how this differed from the picture of insider/outsider divides often painted in the rural literature. Pierce and Scherra had the advantage of having contacted potential subjects through the medical practices in rural areas and thus may have been seen in some manner as an extension of the subject's trusted practitioners. Shreffler (Shreffler, 1999) discussed designing culturally sensitive research methods for surveying rural or frontier residents. This article recommend adapting normal sampling methods by expanding the time frame for survey replies, contacting the local postal department to gain information regarding the best way of addressing mail if addresses are missing from the sampling frame, and preparing for survey research through careful planning and contact with local insiders. Powe and Weinrich (Powe & Weinrich, 1999) described an intervention to decrease fatalism prior to enrolling subjects for a colorectal cancer screening study. These authors identified barriers to participation in research that included cancer screenings of rural, socioeconomically disadvantaged African American elders as including cancer fatalism, lack of knowledge of cancer, poverty, and poor access to health care. This study focused on building upon spirituality to reduce cancer fatalism among these rural elders.

Finally, it might be reasonable to draw information from farm research projects, since many rural dwellers who have participated in research have done so in the form of surveys focused on agricultural issues. One study (Norman et al., 1998) reported that farmers would rather be partners in research than have research done for them, thus lending support for action research methodologies in rural areas.

The current study replicates and extends the work of Trauth et al. (2000). In their review of the literature, they found that there is "an extensive literature regarding willingness to participate in medical research studies from the perspectives of patients being treated for a particular disease, patients who have survived a disease, as well as members of various high risk populations" (p. 25). Trauth et al. (2000) found that certain health and demographic variables were associated with willingness to participate in a medical research study. Respondents with higher income (52%) and more education (50%) were more willing to participate, as were younger respondents. Those with children (43%) were less willing to participate, and gender had no influence on willingness. Respondents who had a close family member who was ill were much more willing to participate (58%), but an illness of their own did not increase likelihood of participation. Prior participation was associated with willingness to participate (55%).

Trauth et al. (2000) separated respondents into groups named "willing," "not willing," and "undecided" in whether they would participate in research. These authors discussed attitudes and knowledge as possibly influencing the decision to participate in a study but did not ask their sample about possible barriers to participation, nor did they sample from a rural population.

## Methods

A survey was developed based on the work of Trauth et al. (2000) with added questions and re-wording. Changes focused on health care research rather than clinical trials or medical research alone and other health care professionals as researchers, in addition to doctors. In addition, questions regarding potential barriers to research participation were added to the survey. The added questions were based on the literature and hypothesized rural influences, such as distance and isolation.

The Binghamton University Human Subjects Research Review Committee approved the research proposal. This was a confidential survey. A sampling frame of 45,000 property owners in Delaware County in upstate New York was obtained from the county tax rolls. Property owners who had out-of-county mailing addresses were removed, and a random sample of households was then chosen using every eighth name on the list. Five thousand surveys consisting of 100 items were mailed in July and August 2002. Subjects were asked if they could be contacted if there was any missing information. Those agreeing to the additional contact were asked to provide a phone number or email address. Approximately 100 calls were made to obtain responses on missing items. This measure increased the pool of usable surveys. Eight hundred and sixty five usable surveys were returned and analyzed.

As surveys were returned, data entry was completed utilizing SPSS software. Data were analyzed to create scales for willingness, attitudes, knowledge, and barriers. The wealth of data provided in the returned surveys on the broad topic of willingness to participate in research does not lend itself to reporting in one article. Barriers to participation in research are often discussed anecdotally in the health care and research literature, but there is a dearth of literature actually examining barriers to participation in research by rural dwellers.

Thus, the focus of this article is the barrier scale developed from 39 items on the survey.

## Description of the Sample

Delaware County, a large county situated in upstate New York, has no metropolitan areas, and the nearest metropolitan area is an average of one hour away by car. The population was 47,520 in 2001. Other characteristics of interest are noted in Table 1 (U.S. Census Bureau, 2003).

**Table 1**
*Population Characteristics of County, State, and United States*

|  | *Delaware County* | *New York State* | *United States* |
|---|---|---|---|
| Population density | 33.2/sq. mile | 401.9/sq. mile | 79.6/sq. mile |
| Persons 65 years and over | 18.6% | 12.9% | 12.4% |
| White persons | 96.4% | 67.9% | 75.1% |
| Home ownership rate | 75.7% | 53.0% | 66.2% |
| Median household income | $32,461 | $43,393 | $41,994 |

Comparison of township population and response rate per township was significant at $p < .000$ ($r = 0.962$). Sixty-four percent of the respondents were female. Young people were under-represented, with 45% of the respondents between the ages of 50 and 69. The high percentage of elders ($\geq 65 = 18.6\%$) in the county was reflected in the responses, as 22% of the respondents were age 70 or over. Forty percent of the sample had always lived in a rural place; likewise, 40% first lived in a city and then moved to a rural place, 18% migrated from rural to urban and back to rural, and three percent currently migrate between urban and rural places.

Not surprisingly, since they responded to this study, most of the participants (95%) were in favor of health care research. Respondents were willing to use tax dollars to support research on health care issues such as cancer (85%) and heart disease (83%). Fewer respondents were willing to have tax dollars used to support the study of depression (68%), alcoholism (61%), and teen pregnancy (55%). However, it should be noted that over half the respondents were at least hypothetically willing to have tax dollars go to research in what to some are less socially acceptable issues. This willingness to support some types of research over others roughly corresponds with the findings of Trauth's et al. (2000). They also found that willingness to participate varied with disease: cancer 88%, heart disease 86%, and depression 78%. Political views and issues of the use of tax dollars may also influence findings in this area but need further exploration.

## Results and Discussion

Based on the literature, thirty-nine items were selected from the survey that might potentially address barriers to research participation. Validity and reliability of the scale were assessed by factor analysis and reliability estimates. Factor analysis is used to determine if items cluster into components or factors that can be interpreted conceptually.

All 39 items were entered into SPSS 13.0 database. The Kaiser-Meyer-Olkin (KMO) measure of sampling adequacy was 0.845, indicating that the item pool is appropriate for factor analysis procedures. Several iterations of factor analysis resulted in a final solution of seven factors containing 29 items that were found to explain 63% of the variance, as seen in Table 2. Item-total analysis and Cronbach's alpha were conducted to create an internally consistent barrier scale consisting of these 29 items, which together had a Cronbach's alpha of 0.81.

In the presence of illness (factor 1), people are more willing to participate in research; however, fatal illness may be conceptualized as a barrier to participation in research. This is supported in the literature, where over 50% of the sample in one study reported they would be unwilling to participate as a subject if they had a fatal illness (Trauth et al., 2000). The intangible benefits (factor 2) retained 5 items which included learning about one's own health, helping the community, and having a convenient research site. Items that made up the convenience factor included low risks, not having to miss work (reverse coded), driving less than 30 minutes for study, and a researcher who did not speak a different language (reverse coded).

Tangible rewards included gifts or other rewards. Trust barriers were not knowing the researcher, not knowing others in the study, and not trusting the researcher. If the study required getting time off from work, or occurred during business hours, it was considered a barrier of timing (factor 6). The Logistics items that remained in the barriers scale after rotations included a lack of money, lack of transportation, and bad driving conditions as barriers to participation.

**Table 2**
*Barrier Scale Factors*

| Factor Number | Factor Name | Variance explained | Cronbach's alpha of factor | No. of items |
|---|---|---|---|---|
| 1 | Illness | 15% | .8864 | 7 |
| 2 | Intangible Benefits | 12% | .8774 | 5 |
| 3 | Convenience | 9% | .7140 | 6 |
| 4 | Tangible Rewards | 8% | .8004 | 3 |
| 5 | Trust | 7% | .7041 | 3 |
| 6 | Timing | 6% | .8207 | 2 |
| 7 | Logistics | 6% | .5199 | 3 |

Although the researchers may conceptualize where an item would fit when putting together a survey, the mathematical formulation of the factors, not the researcher, ultimately decides which items come together to form a factor. For example, having a convenient site at which to participate may logically fit into both the convenience and intangible benefits (factors 2 and 3) in the mind of the researcher, but the after factor analysis this item was found in the intangible benefits factor.

Scores on the barrier scale were inverse. Thus, a high score meant that person perceived fewer barriers then a person who had a low score. This is interpreted to mean that the individual with a lower score had more barriers to participation in research. Scores on the barrier scale ranged from 12 to 60 with a mean ($\mu$) of 35.30 and a standard deviation (SD) of 8.44. Those who were classified as younger, defined as 58 years old (the median age) or less, had significantly lower ($p = 0.00$) barrier scores ($\mu = 34$, SD = 7.8) than those who were older ($\mu = 37$, SD = 8.6) in this study. Males scored significantly lower on the barriers scale than females, indicating more barriers to participation in health care research. These findings may be explained in part by the employment data reported in this sample. The younger ($X^2 = 348$, df = 2, p = 0.00) and male ($X^2 = 13.8$, df = 2, p = 0.001) participants were most likely to report being employed over their older and female counterparts. Those participants living in the most rural areas of the county, with local populations of 2,500 or less, scored significantly higher on the barrier scale (p = 0.00) indicating they perceived fewer barriers to participation than those living in the more populated areas of the county.

Mean barrier scores were calculated for those least willing (33.56), undecided (36.93) and most willing (38.04) to participate in research among this sample. A one-way analysis of variance (ANOVA) was calculated to identify any significant differences in barrier scores by level of willingness to participate in research. The results were statistically significant (F = 18.63, df 2, 808, p = 0.00), indicating that those with the lowest barrier scores, and thus the highest perception of barriers, were among the least willing to participate as research subjects.

## Rural Implications

The specific barriers that are notable for rural areas were transportation issues, work-related issues, and outsider issues. Potential participants desired free transportation, a drive of less than 30 minutes, or would find bad driving conditions a barrier. They would not miss work in order to participate. Finally, if the researcher was unknown or spoke a different language, then respondents would be less likely to participate in research.

When planning a research study, it is important for researchers to know that rural dwellers would be more likely to participate if a convenient site were chosen and season was taken into consideration. Data collection should be done outside of business hours. Response rate would likely be improved by use of local data collectors, known to the potential subjects. Despite the barriers to participation, it appears that residents living in the most rural locations may be accustomed to overcoming barriers such as distance and isolation. They may see these issues as less prohibitive to participation than do those living in more populated areas within a rural county.

Demographic data were examined in relation to scoring on the barrier scale. Men scored lower on the barrier scale than women; as did those younger than 58 years of age (the median age), indicating that men and younger subjects perceived more barriers to participating in research than women or older subjects in this sample.

## Limitations

Obvious sampling limitations in this study were gender, age, and race. In 64% of households, women answered the survey, compared to 66% in Trauth et al. (2000). In this county, there is a high proportion of elders, and the sampling was biased toward older people by using property owners as the mailing database. Similarly, there is lack of racial diversity in this county, and therefore fewer ethnic groups were represented in the sample. A further problem created by using property tax records for mailing was the exclusion of renters, who are typically those who cannot afford homes, younger people, and possibly racial minorities. Generalizability is limited by these sampling concerns.

Some limitations were created by the procedures chosen. For example, there was only one mailing of the survey. Follow-up cards and a second wave of surveys may have increased the return rate, but costs were prohibitive. Another limitation in this sample may have been the timing of the survey, which was mailed in late July and early August. The advantage of this timing was that the survey was more likely to capture those who have a second home in Delaware County, thus adding diversity to the sample. The disadvantage to a summer mailing was that it is possible to miss potential subjects due to vacations during the sampling period. However, we continued to add surveys to the data base anytime they were returned, and some were returned up to three months after the survey. The demographic representativeness of the responses in relation to the population of the county where the data were collected was encouraging, indicating the findings were generalizable to the population in this rural northeast county.

The surveys were self-report without opportunity for verification. While the areas under study were not particularly sensitive, it is still possible that people will answer in a manner to satisfy the researcher.

# Conclusions

Inclusion of rural people in health care research will ultimately have a positive influence in the quality of health care they receive. This study, conducted in a county that demonstrates many common rural features, supports many hypotheses about rural participation in health care research but does not support the idea that rural location alone is a barrier to participation in research. Particular features of rural life have an impact on rural people's willingness to participate in research. However, these concerns can be addressed through research design to improve recruitment. Data from this survey regarding knowledge and attitudes are also being analyzed for their effect on rural people's willingness to participate in health care research.

## NOTES

This project was supported by funding from the O'Connor Office of Rural Health Studies, Decker School of Nursing, Binghamton University.

We also thank the Research Assistants of the O'Connor Office, the McNair Scholars Program, and Faculty of the Decker School of Nursing.

From: Morgan, L. L., Fahs, P. S., & Klesh, J. (2005). Barriers to research participation identified by rural people. *Journal of Agricultural Safety and Health, 11,* 407–414. Copyright 2005 by the American Society of Agricultural Engineers (ASAE). Reprinted with permission.

## REFERENCES

Apolone, G., & Mosconi, P. (2003). Knowledge and opinions about clinical research. *Journal Ambulatory Care Management, 26,* 83–87.

Beck, C. T. (1994). Replication strategies for nursing research. *Image: Journal of Nursing Scholarship, 26*(3), 191–194.

Corbie-Smith, G., Thomas, S., Williams, M., & Moody-Ayers, S. (1999). Attitudes and beliefs of African Americans toward participation in medical research. *Journal of General Internal Medicine, 14,* 537–546.

Daly, J., Sindone, A., Thompson, D., Hancock, K., Chang, E., & Davidson, P. (2002). Barriers to participation in and adherence to cardiac rehabilitation programs: A critical literature review. *Progress in Cardiovascular Nursing, 17,* 8–17.

Ellis, P. (2000). Attitudes towards and participation in randomized clinical trials in oncology: A review of the literature. *Annals of Oncology, 11,* 939–945.

Ellis, P., Butow, P., Simes, R., Tattersall, M., & Dunn, S. (1999). Barriers to participation in randomized clinical trials for early breast cancer among Australian cancer specialists. *The Australian and New Zealand Journal of Surgery, 69*, 486–491.

Fahs, P., Findholt, N., & Daniel, S. (2003). Themes and issues in rural nursing research. In M. Collins (Ed.), *Teaching/learning activities for rural community-based nursing practice* (pp. 56–172). Binghamton, NY: Decker School of Nursing, Binghamton University.

Fallowfield, L., Jenkins, V., Brennan, C., Sawtell, M., Moynihan, C., & Souhami, R. (1998). Attitudes of patients to randomised clinical trials of cancer therapy. *European Journal of Cancer, 10*, 1554–1559.

Fallowfield, L., Ratcliffe, D., & Souhami, R. (1997). Clinician's attitudes to clinical trials of cancer therapy. *European Journal of Cancer, 33*, 2221–2229.

Fisher, P., & Ball, T. (2003). Tribal participatory research: Mechanisms of a collaborative model. *American Journal of Community Psychology, 32*, 207–216.

Grunfeld, E., Zitzelsberger, L., Coristine, M., & Aspelund, F. (2002). Barriers and facilitators to enrollment in cancer clinical trials. *Cancer, 95*, 1577–1583.

Halpern, S., Karlawish, J., Casarett, D., Berlin, J., Townsend, R., & Asch, D. (2003). Hypertensive patient's willingness to participate in placebo-controlled trials: Implications for recruitment efficiency. *American Heart Journal, 146*, 985–992.

Harris, Y., Gorelick, P., Samuels, P., & Bempong, I. (1996). Why African Americans may not be participating in clinical trials. *Journal of the National Medical Association, 88*, 630–634.

Kennedy, B., & Burnett, M. (2002). Clinical research trials: A comparison of African Americans who have and have not participated. *Journal of Cultural Diversity, 9*, 95–97.

Lovato, L., Hill, K., Hertert, S., Hunninghake, D., & Probstfield, J. (1997). Recruitment for controlled clinical trials: Literature summary and annotated bibliography. *Controlled Clinical Trials, 18*, 328–357.

Madsen, S., Mirza, M., Holm, S., Hilsted, K., Kampmann, K., & Riis, P. (2002). Attitudes toward clinical research amongst participants and nonparticipants. *Journal of Internal Medicine, 251*, 156–168.

Maurer, L., Davis, T., Hammond, S., Smith, E., West, P., & Doolittle, M. (2001). Clinical trials in a rural population: Professional education aspects. *Journal of Cancer Education, 16*, 89–92.

Mouton, C., Harris, S., Rovi, S., Solorzano, P., & Johnson, M. (1997). Barriers to black women's participation in cancer clinical trials. *Journal National Medical Association, 89*, 721–727.

Norman, D., Bloomquist, L., Freyenberger, S., Regehr, D., Schurle, B., & Janke, R. (1998). Framers attitudes concerning on-farm research: Kansas survey results. *Journal Natural Resources and Life Sciences Education, 27*, 35–41.

Outlaw, F., Bourjolly, J., & Barg, F. (2000). A study of recruitment of Black Americans into clinical trials through a cultural competence lens. *Cancer Nursing, 23*, 444–451.

Pierce, C., & Scherra, E. (2004). The challenges of data collection in rural dwelling samples. *Online Journal of Rural Nursing and Health Care, 4*(2), Online.

Powe, B., & Weinrich, S. (1999). An intervention to decrease cancer fatalism among rural elders. *Oncology Nursing Forum, 26*, 583–588.

Research!America. (2003). *America speaks poll data.* Alexandria, VA: Author.

Ross, S., Grant, A., Counsell, C., Gillespie, W., Russell, I., & Prescott, R. (1999). Barriers to participation in randomised controlled trials: A systematic review. *Journal of Clinical Epidemiology, 52*, 1143–1156.

Shavers-Hornaday, V., Lynch, C., Burmeister, L., & Torner, J. (1997). Why are African Americans under-represented in medical research studies? Impediments to participation. *Ethnicity and Health, 2*, 31–45.

Shavers, V., Lynch, C., & Burmeister, L. (2000a). Factors that influence African-Americans' willingness to participate in medical research studies. *Cancer, 91*(Supplement), 233–236.

Shavers, V., Lynch, C., & Burmeister, L. (2000b). Knowledge of the Tuskegee study and its impact on the willingness to participate in medical research studies. *Journal of the National Medical Association, 92*, 563–572.

Shreffler, M. (1999). Culturally sensitive research methods of surveying rural/frontier residents. *Western Journal of Nursing Research, 21*, 426–435.

Trauth, J., Musa, D., Siminoff, L., Jewell, I., & Ricci, E. (2000). Public attitudes regarding willingness to participate in medical research studies. *Journal of Health and Social Policy, 12*(2), 23–43.

U.S. Census Bureau. (2003). *American fact finder.* Retrieved October 23, 2003, From http://www.census.gov/

Unson, C., Dunbar, N., Curry, L., Kenyon, L., & Prestwood, K. (2001). The effects of knowledge, attitudes, and significant others on decisions to enroll in a clinical trial on Osteoporosis: Implications for recruitment of older African-American women. *Journal of the National Medical Association, 93*, 392–401.